About the Author

Jananie (Jan) Nallathamby is the director of a renowned consultancy firm in the United Kingdom, which has specialised in finance and business consultancy for over 16 years. Based in London, Jan is celebrated for her adept navigation of intricate financial and tech landscapes, driving remarkable business success.

Jan's journey beyond her professional achievements demonstrates resilience and holistic insight. Confronting the challenges of functional IBS-C disorder, she has gained a profound understanding of the delicate interplay between health and professional life. Jan embodies resilience, and it demonstrates how determination and compassion matter.

Through her writing, Jan offers invaluable insights into balancing personal well-being with professional excellence, drawing from her unique perspective.

When not immersed in consulting, Jan finds joy in diverse passions. Splitting her time between London, India and Sri Lanka, she finds peace through writing, gardening, and enjoying the pleasure of nurturing life in lush greenery. In her spare time, she embarks on thrilling adventures across the globe, is an avid reader and shares a profound connection with horses.

GUT HEALTH GUIDE FOR IBS

A Holistic Approach For All Ages: Tips On Gluten-Onion-Garlic-Free Diet, Mindset, Exercises, Time And Stress Management With Natural Remedies

JAN NALLATHAMBY
ACMA, CGMA, MSc
IBS Lived Expert With Over 25 Years Of Experience

ISBN 979-8-33548-118-2

Printed in the United Kingdom.

I dedicate this book to everyone facing the challenges of functional irritable bowel syndrome (IBS) type C (constipation-predominant). However, the general advice within may be helpful for all types of IBS. With over 25 years of personal experience facing IBS challenges, I empathise deeply with your journey. I stand in solidarity with you, acknowledging the complexities and difficulties you are facing in finding solutions to these ailments. Your resilience, courage, and determination in adversity are genuinely inspiring.

To all who have shared their stories with bravery, your courage lights the way to understanding, empathy, and healing. Your voices echo within these pages, showing the strength in unity, communal support, and empathetic bonds.

May this book be a source of hope and empowerment for all those living with IBS? May it provide comfort during times of uncertainty, clarity in moments of doubt, and motivation to strive for better health and well-being.

Reviews from great customers like you help others feel confident choosing this book. Your positive feedback will be much appreciated. Enjoy the read.

With deepest gratitude and admiration,
Jan Nallathamby

Acknowledgements

I am profoundly grateful to Darlene Fernandes, Judith-Mara Lange, James Hawkins, my family, and friends for their unwavering love, support, motivation, and endless patience during the creation of this book. Your presence in my life is a constant source of inspiration, and I cherish our shared moments.

Note to the reader

As someone who has personally experienced IBS-C, I bring authenticity and credibility to the recommendations in my book. However, it is essential to note that this book does not replace medical advice. Consulting a healthcare professional for symptoms or medical needs is always recommended. The content is based on my personal experiences, as I am not a trained doctor, dietician, or gastro specialist. Therefore, seeking personalised medical guidance and conducting your due diligence is essential. Never stop medication without consulting a doctor.

I only feature products I use and recommend, and unless otherwise noted, the references to services and products are unsponsored. Some of the links included are affiliate links, and I may earn a commission if you purchase them at no additional cost. For more information, visit my additional resources.

It is my sincere hope that this book brings joy and valuable insights to others, just as it has to me. I wish you all the best in your journey to good health and a fulfilling life. Remember, this book is not a replacement for medical advice, but a companion in your quest for better health and well-being.

CONTENTS

Introduction

Embark on a journey to manage Irritable Bowel Syndrome (IBS) naturally with this comprehensive guide, enriched by over 25 years of personal experience dealing with IBS-C (predominant constipation). This book addresses symptoms like abdominal discomfort, bloating, gas, feeling full quickly, weight fluctuations, and constipation, focusing on individuals' sensitivities to gluten, lactose, fructose, onion, and garlic. Understanding how IBS can disrupt social interactions and daily routines, especially for those leading busy lives, provides practical solutions suitable for individuals of all ages and lifestyles globally.

From understanding diagnosis to dietary strategies and lifestyle practices, readers will learn how to optimise their gut health and well-being. The inclusion of future research directions in this guide provides hope for ongoing improvement, instilling a sense of optimism in the readers.

This book is a beacon of simplicity and practicality, designed to assist both new and long-term IBS-C individuals. The general tips apply to all types of IBS. It offers holistic advice for gradually improving IBS symptoms without promoting instant solutions. It provides solutions catering to various budgets and avoids technical jargon, ensuring easy understanding for all readers without medical backgrounds. It covers psychological approaches to diet-based and holistic methods with meal tips and tricks rather than complex recipes, catering to plant and meat eaters.

Ultimately, this book is designed to empower readers to take control of their gut health and live well despite the challenges of IBS-C. It encourages readers to experiment with new approaches and adopt a positive mindset to enhance their quality of life at home and work. This book aims to guide those with IBS-C towards an optimal lifestyle, putting the power back in the readers' hands. However, since everyone is different, individual dietary intolerances should be considered.

My IBS-C journey

During my 25-year journey with IBS-M (with mixed symptoms of both constipation and diarrhoea), which began in my school years and transitioned to IBS-C, I have gained significant insights. Despite the absence of any family history, it is possible that job-related stress played a role in my development of IBS-C in a way that highlights the importance of maintaining a balanced lifestyle. Initially, I consulted my doctor and joined a study at King's College London, adopting the low FODMAP (Fermentable Oligosaccharides, Disaccharides, Monosaccharides, and Polyols) diet to identify triggers such as gluten, lactose, spicy and gassy foods, onions, garlic, fructose, and coffee. This posed challenges in social situations. Despite benefits, I faced weight fluctuations, nutrient deficiencies, and constipation, highlighted by MRI and blood tests ruling out coeliac disease. I have bolstered my gut health and feel more energised by attending regular online IBS sessions and maintaining a daily routine of probiotic tablets containing 20 billion gut-friendly bacteria for over a year. I am on a three-month break from the probiotic tablet, following advice from the pharmacy before I resume. As further research on the gut microbiome develops, I maintain a positive outlook during periods of experimentation.

What is IBS?

IBS is a common long-term digestive disorder affecting the large intestine, not caused by food allergies. It is classified as a functional gastrointestinal disorder, indicating it involves communication between the brain and gut. IBS is persistent and can last for years, with symptoms that can come and go and often worsen as individuals get older. These symptoms include abdominal discomfort, cramping, bloating, gas, and changes in bowel habits like diarrhoea, constipation, or both.

Research suggests that IBS affects about 5-10% of people worldwide, making it one of the most prevalent gastrointestinal disorders. It has been known by different names in the past, like nervous colon or spastic bowel.

While IBS does not shorten life expectancy, it can significantly affect quality of life. Individuals with IBS often find it challenging to manage social situations and work responsibilities because of the unpredictable nature of their symptoms. For instance, they might have to leave meetings unexpectedly, skip certain foods at social gatherings, experience discomfort in their lower abdomen when sitting for extended periods at work or often need to use the restroom. These situations make planning ahead tricky and can cause stress and anxiety. Raising awareness about these challenges at home and work is essential, which is why IBS Awareness Month is in April. This helps promote understanding and support for those living with this condition.

IBS by gender

Research has shown that the occurrence of IBS differs between genders. For example, a study in "Digestive Diseases and Sciences" in 2021 estimated that IBS affects about 10-15% of women. Another study published in "Gastroenterology" in 2019 discovered that women are twice as likely as men to develop IBS. According to the National Institute of Diabetes and Digestive and Kidney Diseases (NIDDK), women are more prone to symptoms like abdominal discomfort, diarrhoea, and constipation compared to men. Even though men are less likely to have IBS, they may experience more severe symptoms if they do. Moreover, men tend to seek medical help less often for IBS symptoms than women do.

It is essential to understand that IBS is a long-term condition that can affect individuals of all ages. However, it is often diagnosed more frequently in individuals between 20 and 50. Since IBS appears in various studies, there is a need for more research to better understand gut health and improve management for those affected.

IBS can occur at any age but often develops in early adulthood. However, it is also common for symptoms to appear later in life, including after age 50. Older adults may experience changes in bowel habits, abdominal discomfort, and bloating. Getting advice from a medical professional can effectively help manage symptoms.

While IBS-C affects both genders, there may be differences in how it manifests. Research generally indicates that women are more frequently diagnosed with IBS, including IBS-C.

Some studies suggest that women with IBS-C might have more severe symptoms during menstruation due to hormonal changes, like abdominal discomfort and bloating. They may also be susceptible to conditions like endometriosis or pelvic floor dysfunction, which can worsen symptoms.

However, these differences aren't absolute, and both genders can experience a variety of symptoms and severity levels with IBS-C. Treatment typically involves dietary adjustments, stress management, and sometimes medication, regardless of gender.

IBS in children and during pregnancy

Children aged 4 to 18 years old are also affected by IBS, with rates estimated at 5-10%. Symptoms vary, including abdominal pain, diarrhoea, and constipation. Creating a supportive environment, consistent meals, and toilet routines can help. Identifying trigger foods and collaborating with a healthcare provider for a tailored diet plan is crucial. Teaching relaxation techniques and providing reassurance would help manage stress and anxiety. Consulting a paediatrician or gastroenterologist ensures specialised care.

According to the U.S. National Institutes of Health, IBS can develop during or after pregnancy due to hormonal, stress, dietary, and physical changes. Managing symptoms during pregnancy involves a balanced diet with fibre-rich foods, hydration, small frequent meals, and stress reduction. Lifestyle changes such as exercise and fibre-rich diets aid in preventing constipation. Avoiding triggers and seeking medical guidance ensures a healthier pregnancy.

While IBS typically does not directly affect the baby, managing symptoms is vital. Severe symptoms like diarrhoea or constipation can lead to complications like dehydration or nutrient deficiencies if left untreated. Collaborating with healthcare providers ensures a safe maternal and foetal health management plan during pregnancy.

Safe laxatives and stool softeners can help with constipation during pregnancy, but they should be used with a doctor's supervision. Iron supplements may also cause constipation in pregnant women; therefore, informing your healthcare provider about any iron supplements you are taking can help manage constipation.

Different types of IBS

Each subtype of IBS comes with its symptoms and management challenges, necessitating tailored approaches for relief and improved quality of life:

1. IBS-D (IBS with diarrhoea): shows frequent diarrhoea episodes, often with abdominal discomfort and urgency.
2. IBS-C (IBS with constipation): features infrequent bowel movements and difficulty passing stool, alongside abdominal discomfort or bloating.
3. IBS-M (mixed IBS): presents a mix of symptoms, including both diarrhoea and constipation, alternating or occurring together.
4. PI-IBS (post-infectious IBS): this condition emerges after a gastrointestinal infection and results in ongoing IBS symptoms after recovery.
5. IBS-U (unspecified IBS): applied when symptoms do not neatly fit into other subtypes or fluctuate over time.

IBS symptoms

Personal insights: the triggers for IBS can change with age. Staying active and maintaining a positive mindset can help manage symptoms. Still, it is different for everyone, and there is no guarantee. Listening to and working with your body is essential to find what works for you.

Often, a mix of symptoms arises without visible damage or disease in the digestive tract. These include recurring abdominal pain and changes in bowel movements, like diarrhoea, constipation, or both. Constipation means having three or fewer bowel movements per week or having difficulty passing them (IBS-C). Diarrhoea involves loose, watery, or frequent bowel movements. Additional symptoms may include bloating, gas, or urgency (IBS-D).

Common IBS symptoms include:

- Abdominal discomfort and cramps
- Bloating is often experienced more by women and can feel like swelling, tightness, or hardness in the abdomen. It is frequently seen in functional disorders like severe IBS, worsening throughout the day, and may not change with gynaecological problems.
- Gas
- Diarrhoea
- Constipation
- Alternating diarrhoea and constipation
- Presence of mucus in the stool
- Fatigue
- Difficulty sleeping

These symptoms result from the irregular movement of food through the intestines. Excessive speed can lead to diarrhoea, and sluggishness can lead to constipation. Increased sensitivity of abdominal nerves to pain also contributes to discomfort. In some cases, symptoms are made worse by eating.

IBS is characterised by two main elements:

1. An abdominal discomfort that is either relieved by defaecation or
2. Alterations in bowel habits, including changes in stool texture and frequency (straining, urgency, incomplete evacuation).

Non-colon-related IBS symptoms

Non-colon-related symptoms of IBS, known as extracolonic symptoms, can vary widely and include fatigue, headaches, muscle pain, sleep disturbances, urinary frequency, sexual dysfunction, anxiety, depression, nausea, heartburn, joint pain, skin issues like eczema, and cognitive difficulties such as brain fog. These symptoms may not always directly correlate with gastrointestinal problems and can differ in intensity among individuals.

Short episodes of high temperature after consuming gluten may indicate a sensitivity or intolerance, often associated with conditions like coeliac disease. Other high FODMAP triggers like onions and garlic may also need to be avoided. IBS-C can present neurological (headaches, dizziness, and difficulty concentrating), endocrine (hormonal fluctuations and thyroid abnormalities), cardiovascular (heart palpitations), and respiratory (shortness of breath) symptoms, which may occur alongside or independently of gastrointestinal issues.

Recognising and addressing these symptoms is essential for holistic management. Despite the physical toll, the emotional and psychological impact of IBS should not be overlooked. The stigma surrounding digestive disorders can prevent individuals from seeking help, perpetuating their combat.

Causes of IBS

There can be multiple causes for IBS, making it critical to identify the underlying factors for effective treatment.

Common causes include:

1. Stress (most prevalent): related to life events or work pressures.
2. Dietary habits: irregular meals, excessive caffeine, alcohol consumption, or indulgence in fatty and sugary foods.

The exact cause of IBS remains a mystery, but several factors might play a role in its development. Researchers are looking into how our gut and brain communicate with each other and how changes in the bacteria living in our gut might be linked to IBS.

If you are under a lot of stress, whether from work or personal life, it could make you more likely to develop IBS. Stress can mess with the way our gut and brain talk to each other.

Eating lots of processed foods and needing more fibre might increase your chances of getting IBS. Fibre is good for gut bacteria, so insufficient can disturb your digestive system.

If you have food allergies or other allergies, they could cause inflammation in your gut, which might lead to IBS symptoms.

Getting a stomach bug or other gut infections can cause inflammation in the gut, too, which could contribute to IBS.

Having surgery on your stomach, especially on the intestines, can sometimes increase the risk of IBS because it can mess with the nerves and muscles in your gut.

Those with IBS often have sensitivity issues with the muscles and nerves in their intestines, which can lead to pain, cramps, and diarrhoea.

Sometimes, the balance of good and bad bacteria in our guts gets disrupted, and that imbalance can irritate our intestines.

Having a family history of IBS or other mental health conditions such as anxiety or depression can also heighten the likelihood of developing IBS. Factors like Crohn's disease or ulcerative colitis can raise your chances of getting IBS. Sometimes, individuals with IBS also have other related problems like functional dyspepsia or constipation. Dyspepsia is upper abdominal discomfort, heartburn, feeling full quickly, bloating, nausea, and belching.

Common IBS triggers

Include and not limited to:

Certain foods like lactose in dairy, gluten in wheat, and specific fermentable carbohydrates in beans can lead to bloating and discomfort. Gluten, an IBS trigger, is a protein found in wheat, barley and rye, commonly in bread, pasta, pizza, sauces, cakes, and more. It lends elasticity to dough, aiding in bread rising and creating soft textures. This book also highlights onion and garlic intolerance. Millions globally grapple with gluten, fructose and lactose intolerance, experiencing symptoms like discomfort, bloating, headaches, and more.

Stress disrupts the connection between your gut (digestive system) and brain, leading to intensified IBS symptoms such as abdominal discomfort, bloating, and irregular bowel movements.

Caffeine stimulates the gut, causing increased bowel movements and potentially exacerbating IBS symptoms like diarrhoea and abdominal pain.

Alcohol can inflame the gut lining and disrupt digestion, which can worsen IBS symptoms like pain and bloating.

Smoking affects gut function and blood flow, accelerating symptoms like pain and discomfort.

During menstruation, as hormone levels decrease, symptoms such as stomach pain, discomfort, and alternating constipation or diarrhoea may intensify.

While there is no known cure for IBS, I have discovered that it can be managed effectively over the years. Adopting the tips in this book could help you manage your condition better and enjoy a higher quality of life.

Irritable Bowel Syndrome

"Maybe you are searching among the branches, for what only appears in the roots." — Rumi

In a normal gut, digestion occurs smoothly, with food passing through the digestive system without causing discomfort or irregular bowel movements. The gut microbiome, consisting of a diverse community of beneficial bacteria, helps maintain gut health by aiding digestion and nutrient absorption.

Conversely, a dysfunctional gut, such as in individuals with IBS, experiences disruptions in digestion and gut function. This can cause symptoms such as abdominal pain, bloating, gas, diarrhoea, or constipation. Factors like imbalances in gut bacteria, heightened gut sensitivity or abnormalities in gut motility can contribute to these disturbances, leading to discomfort and affecting overall well-being. Understanding the differences between normal and abnormal gut is crucial for effectively identifying and managing gastrointestinal conditions.

1. Diagnosis

"Be the sun and all will see you." — Fyodor Dostoevsky

IBS-C is not yet fully understood, and no definitive diagnostic tests or one-size-fits-all treatment exist. Diagnosis is typically determined based on a person's symptoms and detailed medical history. While it can be challenging to manage, dietary and lifestyle changes can significantly improve symptoms for many individuals. It is vital to receive a confirmed diagnosis of IBS and rule out other conditions like coeliac disease and IBD.

For those new to IBS, the diagnosis can be overwhelming. Books tailored to beginners provide essential information, explaining symptoms, triggers, and management strategies. These resources assist individuals in managing their health by offering reassurance and guidance during confusing and frustrating times. Diagnosing the condition typically involves a comprehensive evaluation of symptoms, a detailed medical history, and sometimes diagnostic tests for confirmation. Healthcare providers may rely on the Rome IV criteria, a set of guidelines for diagnosing IBS, to identify recurring abdominal pain, discomfort, and other symptoms.

For those who have been dealing with IBS for a long time, the diagnosis might follow a similar path but with an emphasis on tracking symptom patterns over time and assessing the success of past management techniques. Healthcare providers may also consider the person's medical background and any prior tests or treatments for IBS.

Managing the subtleties of this condition and its symptoms can be difficult. Yet, trusted resources such as books authored by reputable experts offer valuable guidance, aiding in exploring treatment choices and adjustments to one's lifestyle. It is essential to remain open to continuous learning, as new insights may offer fresh strategies for symptom management, bringing hope for an improved quality of life.

Diagnostic criteria

The diagnosis of IBS-C is primarily symptom-based and follows established guidelines such as the Rome IV criteria, the latest version published in 2016, which provides a standardised approach. It indicates that diagnosing IBS-C requires abdominal pain or discomfort to occur at least one day per week over the past three months, along with two or more of the following criteria:
- Improvement in the ease of bowel movements
- The onset is linked to a change in how often stools occur
- Change in the form or appearance of stool

Therefore, if an individual presents with these symptoms, it is advisable to consult a healthcare professional for further evaluation and diagnosis confirmation, as these criteria serve as a guide to identifying and managing IBS-C effectively. It is crucial to consult your doctor to rule out other possible causes for your symptoms, such as celiac disease, Crohn's disease, and cancer.

Medical evaluation

1. Medical history: a detailed history of symptoms, bowel habits, dietary patterns, and medical conditions.
2. Physical examination: a thorough one may reveal abdominal tenderness, bloating, or other signs suggestive of IBS-C.
3. Diagnostic tests:
   - Blood tests: these screen for conditions like coeliac disease or thyroid disorders.
   - Stool sample analysis: the doctor provides a container for testing stool samples for blood or signs of infections.
   - Rectal exam: checks for constipation, rectal tenderness, and other issues during a physical exam.
   - Imaging studies: sometimes, a colonoscopy or abdominal ultrasound may be recommended to rule out structural abnormalities.
   - Other tests: additional tests, such as lactose intolerance tests or breath tests for small intestinal bacterial overgrowth (SIBO), may be considered based on clinical suspicion.

After a detailed medical history assessment, a comprehensive understanding of IBS-C can be achieved, guiding effective management strategies.

Differential diagnosis

It is essential to get an official IBS diagnosis and ensure other conditions like coeliac disease, unexplained weight loss, family history of bowel or ovarian cancer or IBD are ruled out. It is essential to differentiate IBS-C from other gastrointestinal disorders with similar symptoms, including:
- Chronic constipation: characterised by infrequent bowel movements without abdominal pain.
- Inflammatory Bowel Disease (IBD) presents with symptoms like abdominal pain, diarrhoea, and rectal bleeding.
- Functional constipation: similar to IBS-C but lacks the characteristic abdominal discomfort.
- Diagnosing IBS-C requires a systematic approach, integrating symptom assessment, medical history review, and appropriate diagnostic tests. Accurate diagnosis is fundamental for initiating targeted management strategies and improving patient outcomes.

2. Understanding Individual Variations in IBS

"I do not believe anything very certainly, but everything very probably." — Christiaan Huygens

Symptoms vary in severity for each person, and ongoing research seeks targeted solutions as of 2024. Understanding the individual variations in Irritable Bowel Syndrome with constipation (IBS-C) is vital for personalised management and improved quality of life. This chronic gastrointestinal disorder manifests differently among individuals, with symptoms ranging from constipation and abdominal discomfort to bloating, gas, or rectal urgency. Triggers for symptoms vary widely, including dietary choices, stress levels, and lifestyle habits. Tailoring management strategies to address specific triggers is essential for minimising symptom flare-ups. Treatment options vary from non-prescription medications to prescription drugs that target muscular overactivity in the digestive system and hypersensitivity. By considering factors such as symptom severity, triggers, and treatment response, healthcare providers play a crucial role in optimising care for individuals with IBS, providing the support and understanding you need.

Understanding your IBS condition can help you manage it better. With guidance from doctors, you can stick to treatment plans effectively. However, it is also important to remember that you are not alone in this journey. Seeking educational resources and support groups can significantly improve outcomes for those with IBS, providing a sense of connection and community. Ongoing efforts to find new ways to help you manage IBS more effectively show a commitment to finding better solutions. By learning more about IBS and connecting with others who share your experience, you can take control and improve your quality of life.

In Ayurveda, health is influenced by three energies called doshas: Vata, Pitta, and Kapha. When these doshas become imbalanced, it can lead to health issues, including IBS. We will explore how these imbalances relate to IBS.

CHAPTER RECAP:

This chapter explains IBS and how it is diagnosed. IBS causes problems with digestion, leading to symptoms like stomach pain, bloating, and irregular bowel movements. Doctors diagnose IBS based on symptoms and medical history, as no one is still tested for it. Newcomers to IBS might need clarification on the diagnosis, but beginner-friendly books can help. Diagnosis involves checking symptoms, history, and sometimes doing tests like blood or imaging tests like colonoscopy or abdominal ultrasound.

To diagnose IBS properly, doctors follow the Rome IV criteria, which outline symptom patterns for IBS. They might also perform different tests, such as physical exams, blood tests, stool sample checks, and imaging tests, to rule out other problems.

It is essential to tell IBS apart from similar conditions like chronic constipation, IBD, and functional constipation. A correct diagnosis helps find suitable tailored ways to manage IBS and improve individuals' feelings.

Each person's IBS is different, so finding personalised ways to manage it is essential. Symptoms can vary, and things like diet and stress can affect them. Finding ways to manage these triggers can help reduce symptoms. Treatments can range from simple medications to more robust therapies that target the functioning of the gut. Educating individuals about IBS helps them take control of their health. At the same time, ongoing research looks for better ways to help those with IBS.

3. Potential Impact of Body Types on IBS

"I can't go back to yesterday, because I was a different person then." — Lewis Carroll

The ancient Indian medical system of Ayurveda states that there are three doshas, "Vata," "Pitta," and "Kapha," which are the three bioenergies that govern various functions within the body, such as physical, mental, and emotional health. "Ayu" means Life, and " Veda" means knowledge. Each person typically has a unique combination of the three doshas, referred to as their "Prakriti," or constitution.

With a quick 10-minute free survey Dosha Quiz | Discover Your Ayurvedic Body Type | Banyan Botanicals, you can discover your body type using the Dosha quiz link above. **Note:** for full web links mentioned throughout this book, please refer to the chapter 'Additional Resources'. After taking the quiz, you will receive advice on customised meals and lifestyle from Banyan. Their products are not affiliated with or sponsored; the advice will not replace your registered Ayurvedic practitioner. **Tip:** use the dosha quiz often, especially when you are experiencing health issues or imbalances, such as during menstruation, when hormone fluctuations can trigger IBS symptoms. It can help identify potential root causes and offer a comprehensive understanding of your body-mind constitution, supporting overall well-being for those with IBS. **Tip:** tracking your menstruation dates on your mobile phone calendar can help maintain regularity and manage IBS symptoms, as hormonal fluctuations and stress during menstruation can aggravate IBS symptoms.

The doshas in the body are explained further below:

The Vata dosha is associated with elements of air and ether (space), and when balanced, individuals with a dominant Vata constitution tend to have qualities such as creativity, flexibility, and enthusiasm. Pitta dosha is linked to fire and water elements. It is associated with qualities like intelligence, ambition, and determination when in balance. Kapha dosha is associated with earth and water elements, and those with a dominant Kapha constitution often have qualities such as stability, patience, and strength when balanced.

In Ayurvedic medicine, individuals are often categorised based on their dominant dosha or combination of doshas. Here is a brief overview of how each dosha may manifest in terms of body type:

1. Vata body type:
   - Characteristics: generally lean, with a lighter frame and prominent joints.
   - Tendency: prone to fluctuations in weight and digestion.
   - Common symptoms: constipation, gas, bloating, and irregular appetite.
2. Pitta body type:
   - Characteristics: moderate build, with a well-defined musculature.
   - Tendency: can have a moderate appetite and digestion.
   - Common symptoms: acid reflux, heartburn, inflammation, and sensitive digestion.
3. Kapha body type:
   - Characteristics: solid and sturdy build, often with a tendency towards weight gain.
   - Tendency: may have a slower metabolism and digestion.
   - Common symptoms: sluggish digestion, excess mucus, congestion, and water retention.

The imbalances in these doshas are thought to play a role in various health problems, including digestive issues such as IBS. However, it is essential to approach Ayurvedic concepts while considering their cultural and historical context. This encourages appreciation for its holistic approach to health and allows for respectful integration into modern healthcare practices, ensuring the preservation and dissemination of its wisdom for future generations.

While Ayurveda does not directly correlate specific doshas with specific gastrointestinal conditions like IBS-C, it provides insights into how these doshas' imbalances may contribute to digestive disturbances.

For individuals with a dominant Vata constitution, imbalances in Vata dosha may lead to symptoms such as irregular bowel movements, gas, bloating, and dryness in the intestines, which could worsen symptoms of IBS-C.

Likewise, imbalances in Pitta dosha may result in heightened inflammation and irritation within the gastrointestinal tract, which could exacerbate symptoms of IBS-C, such as abdominal discomfort and irregular bowel movements.

For those with a dominant Kapha constitution, imbalances in Kapha dosha may lead to sluggish digestion and metabolism, contributing to symptoms of IBS-C such as constipation and heaviness in the abdomen.

Spicy foods can raise body heat and sometimes cause bloating. Factors like your surroundings when travelling and specific situations, like stress or changes in diet, can also affect IBS symptoms. Consider various factors like these when switching from home remedies to medications.

It is important to note that Ayurveda considers individualised treatment based on a person's unique constitution and imbalances. Therefore, managing IBS-C in Ayurveda would involve restoring balance to the doshas through personalised dietary and lifestyle recommendations, natural remedies, over-prescribed medicines, and practices like yoga and meditation. Consulting with a qualified Ayurvedic practitioner can help tailor treatment to address the specific imbalances contributing to an individual's symptoms of IBS-C. This is further explained in the chapter' Microbiome-Friendly Foods and Recipes'.

Ayurveda and IBS-C

Ayurveda treats everyone individually, focusing on their unique constitution and imbalances. IBS-C aims to balance the doshas through personalised diet and lifestyle changes, using natural remedies when possible, and incorporating practices like yoga and meditation. A qualified Ayurvedic practitioner can tailor treatment to your specific needs. You will find more details in the Microbiome-Friendly Foods and Recipes chapter.

Ayurveda's approach to IBS-C involves diet, lifestyle, and natural remedies. Some specific examples include:

1. Diet changes:
   An Ayurvedic practitioner might suggest a diet based on your dosha. For instance, individuals with a Vata imbalance might receive recommendations to consume warm, moist foods and avoid dry, cold foods that could exacerbate symptoms.
2. Herbal remedies:
   Common Ayurvedic herbs, such as Triphala, which is a mix of three fruits named Amalaki, Bibhitaki, and Haritaki, help digestion and relieve constipation. Another example is tea made from cumin, coriander, and fennel seeds, which also support digestion.
3. Yoga and meditation:
   Certain yoga poses and meditation techniques help manage stress, a common trigger for IBS-C. For example, child's pose (Balasana) and cat-cow stretch (Marjaryasana-Bitilasana) promote digestion and reduce stress. Mindfulness meditation can help manage anxiety, which often makes IBS worse.
4. Example case study for illustration purposes only:
   Manuja, a 35-year-old with a Vata-Pitta constitution, had chronic constipation and bloating. Her Ayurvedic practitioner suggested she eat cooked vegetables and grains, avoiding cold and raw foods. She also drank Triphala and ginger tea before bed. After six months, Manuja felt much better, with fewer symptoms and less stress.
5. Practitioner sample insight:
   Dr Sharda Ayurveda, India's leading Ayurvedic clinic, focuses on balancing the doshas with specific diets and herbs. For example, drinking herbal lukewarm water and adding cow's ghee to one's diet can soothe the digestive system. Gentle yoga and breathing exercises (Pranayama) aid in relieving the mind and enhancing digestion. Aloe vera juice can reduce constipation and diarrhoea by combating bacteria and reducing gut inflammation. Drinking it regularly can ease stomach pain, reduce bloating, and help manage IBS. Please ensure you receive a prescription from a certified Ayurvedic doctor, as treatments would vary for each person based on their doshas, medical conditions and various other factors.

CHAPTER RECAP:

This chapter explored Ayurvedic principles and how they relate to IBS management. Ayurveda identifies three doshas: Vata, Pitta, and Kapha. These doshas influence our body's constitution and health. Understanding our dominant dosha can help tailor dietary and lifestyle practices to promote balance.

Imbalances in these doshas can contribute to digestive issues like IBS. For instance, Vata imbalances may lead to irregular bowel movements. In contrast, Pitta imbalances might cause inflammation and irritation in the gut, leading to discomfort. Kapha imbalances could result in slow digestion and constipation.

Ayurvedic treatment for IBS focuses on restoring doshic balance through personalised dietary adjustments, natural remedies, and practices like yoga and meditation. Consulting with an Ayurvedic practitioner can provide tailored strategies to address individual symptoms and imbalances, leading to holistic healing of IBS symptoms.

Gut Microbiome

"You must have your heart on fire and your brain on ice." — Vladimir Lenin

This chapter discusses the gut microbiome and its impact on health, especially for those with IBS.

First, it explains the gut microbiome, which comprises billions of bacteria and other microorganisms in the human digestive tract. These microorganisms play a pivotal role in keeping the digestive system healthy.

The gut microbiome is a bustling community of tiny organisms in our digestive system. It includes bacteria, fungi, viruses, and other tiny microorganisms. These residents are influenced by our diet, lifestyle, environment, and genes. They play a vital role in keeping our digestive system healthy by helping with digestion, supporting our immune system, and producing critical essential nutrients like vitamins B12 and K and short-chain fatty acids. When the equilibrium of these microorganisms in our gut is disturbed, it can result in issues such as IBS, underscoring the importance of maintaining gut health.

4. Exploring the Microbiome

"It is hard to fight desire; but to control it is the sign of a reasonable man." — Democritus

The chapter discusses the role of the microbiome in digestive health. A healthy gut microbiome is a powerful ally, helping to prevent constipation and diarrhoea, reduce inflammation, and protect against digestive disorders like IBS and coeliac disease. It also improves nutrient absorption by breaking down nutrients, making them easier for the body to use for essential functions and growth.

Next, it covers microbiome dysbiosis in IBS. Dysbiosis indicates an imbalance in the gut microbiome, where the microbial community deviates from its healthy state. It is characterised by excess harmful bacteria and a reduction in beneficial ones. This imbalance can cause symptoms like bloating, abdominal pain, and irregular bowel movements, common for those with IBS. Managing dysbiosis is essential for reducing these symptoms and improving overall gut health.

In summary, this chapter underscores the importance of the gut microbiome in maintaining digestive health and how disturbances in its balance can contribute to symptoms of IBS. It also highlights that understanding and managing the gut microbiome is not just beneficial, but crucial to maintaining a healthy digestive system. This knowledge empowers us to take control of our health and well-being.

5. What is the Gut Microbiome?

"It's amazing how lovely common things become, if one only knows how to look at them." – Louisa May Alcott

The gut microbiome comprises a varied and intricate network of trillions of microorganisms residing within the digestive tract, predominantly found in the large intestine. These microorganisms include bacteria, archaea, fungi, viruses, and protozoa, each playing a pivotal role in maintaining your health. The gut microbiota refers to microorganisms inhabiting the gastrointestinal tract.

Each of us has a unique composition of microbes influenced by diet, lifestyle, environment, and genetics. These small inhabitants play a crucial role in your overall health, including digestion, training your immune system to recognise harmful substances for immunity, nutrient production like vitamins B12 and K, and short-chain fatty acids for gut cell health and fight harmful bacteria. Research hints at a gut microbiome linked to mental conditions like anxiety and depression. Eating disorders, in addition to IBS, can make it challenging to manage IBS symptoms and worsen digestive discomfort, emphasising the importance of comprehensive body and mind care. Chronic stress can negatively impact the microbiome.

This complex interplay highlights the importance of maintaining a healthy gut environment for well-being. Recent studies have shown that a diverse gut microbiome is linked to better overall health. Reduced diversity in the gut microbiome may compromise the immune system, making you more susceptible to infections and illnesses.

The gut microbiome metabolises certain medications, which can impact their effectiveness and safety. This means an individual's gut microbiome can influence how well they respond to specific treatments.

6. Role of the Microbiome in Digestive Health

"A child is not a vase to be filled, but a fire to be lit." — Francois Rabelais

An optimal digestive health relies on a healthy gut microbiome. It helps to:
- **Prevent constipation and diarrhoea** by supporting regular bowel movements and preserving a balanced gut bacteria environment.
- **Reduce inflammation** by producing anti-inflammatory compounds and suppressing the growth of harmful bacteria.
- **Protect against digestive disorders** such as IBS, IBD, and coeliac disease.
- **Improve nutrient absorption** by breaking down nutrients and making them more readily available to the body.

The gut-brain axis in individuals with IBS

The gut houses its own nervous system, the enteric nervous system, communicating with the brain via the spinal cord through the gut-brain axis. This axis influences both physiological and psychological functions, crucial in managing IBS symptoms, supported by evidence-based research as it affects symptom manifestation.

A profound connection exists between the gut and the brain, with the gut's microbiome influencing mood, cognition, and stress response. Individuals with IBS often experience heightened sensitivity to gut signals, leading to increased pain perception. Psychological factors like stress, anxiety, and depression can exacerbate symptoms by amplifying gut-brain interactions. Brain imaging studies have shown altered pain processing in individuals with IBS, even without structural abnormalities in the gut. Innovative approaches like gut-directed hypnotherapy and mindfulness-based stress reduction target this axis to reduce symptoms, providing holistic management for IBS. An **interesting fact:** the gut-brain axis contains more neurotransmitters than the brain, highlighting its significance in regulating mood and emotions. Follow your gut instinct as it is like a second brain, with its hundred trillion bacteria sending signals faster than your central brain.

Interactions between the gut and the central nervous system significantly influence the development and progression of IBS. The pathophysiology of IBS refers to the underlying biological processes that contribute to the growth and manifestation of the condition. It encompasses a complex interaction of various factors, including altered gut motility, visceral hypersensitivity, abnormal gut microbiota composition, immune system dysfunction, and disturbances in the gut-brain axis. These factors can result in symptoms such as abdominal pain, bloating, gas and bowel movements, which characterise IBS. Chronic stress, anxiety, and depression can increase symptom severity and contribute to the cycle of gut-brain interaction and psychological factors like health anxiety, or an illness anxiety disorder can amplify visceral hypersensitivity and provoke levels of stress or worry about their symptom.

Certain beneficial bacteria in the gut also produce neurotransmitters called serotonin, which can affect mood and mental health. This highlights the gut-brain connection.

Studies have shown that the brain's response to pain is altered in individuals with IBS. Functional brain imaging has demonstrated increased activity in brain regions responsible for processing pain signals, like the anterior cingulate cortex and the insula. This overactivity in pain processing regions may contribute to the perception of pain in individuals with IBS, even in the absence of identifiable structural abnormalities in the gut.

Innovative research in this field explores novel approaches to managing IBS symptoms by targeting the gut-brain connection alongside cognitive behaviour therapy and breathing techniques.

CHAPTER RECAP:

This chapter explains the gut microbiome, its importance, and the gut-brain connection in managing IBS.

An optimised digestive health relies significantly on maintaining a healthy gut microbiome. This prevents constipation and diarrhoea by keeping bowel movements regular and balancing gut bacteria. It also reduces inflammation and protects against disorders like IBS and coeliac disease.

The gut and brain communicate via the gut-brain axis, which influences physical and mental functions. This connection affects how IBS symptoms appear and are managed. Individuals with IBS often feel more sensitive to gut signals, making pain worse. Stress and anxiety can intensify these symptoms.

Studies show that IBS patients' brains respond differently to pain. Areas that process pain, like the anterior cingulate cortex and insula, are more active. This might explain why those with IBS feel more pain.

New research is looking at managing IBS by targeting the gut-brain connection. Treatments like gut-directed hypnotherapy and mindfulness-based stress reduction help calm this communication, offering more holistic management of IBS.

Understanding the microbiome and gut-brain axis is crucial in managing IBS. A healthy microbiome supports digestion and protects against disorders, while the gut-brain connection affects symptom management. New treatments focusing on these areas offer hope for better managing IBS.

7. Understanding Microbiome Dysbiosis in IBS

"The less said the better." — Jane Austen

In healthy individuals, a diverse gut microbiome is crucial for digestion and overall well-being. However, in IBS, dysbiosis, or imbalance, can lead to an overabundance of specific microbial groups and a depletion of others. This imbalance impacts the overall metabolic capacity of the gut bacteria, leading to symptoms like bloating and abdominal pain. Understanding and restoring this microbial balance is key. Measures such as reducing processed sugars and stress can help support a healthier gut microbiome. Tracking IBS symptoms and bowel movements using the trackers mentioned in the chapter' Dietary Changes: Meal Planning' can help individuals understand their unique microbiome dysbiosis and identify potential triggers.

In IBS, altered microbial metabolism leads to a complex interplay of factors such as reduced production of beneficial metabolites like short-chain fatty acids, escalated production of harmful metabolites like hydrogen sulfide, changes in gut barrier function, and immune system activation. These interconnected changes contribute to developing and progressing IBS symptoms, impacting gut function, inflammation, and overall well-being.

Several factors, such as diet, stress, genetics, medications, and factors in early life and other influences, can disrupt the fragile balance of the gut microbiota, resulting in diverse health issues and heightened intestinal permeability. This results in harmful substances leaking into the bloodstream, triggering inflammation and contributing to IBS symptoms. IBS can be painful, but it usually does not cause other serious health problems or damage the digestive tract. However, ongoing research may provide new insights.

Important: unless your doctor explicitly recommends them, medications like antibiotics can harm the balance of good bacteria in your gut, which is important for keeping your digestion healthy. Gut bacteria can produce metabolites that influence brain-gut communication, potentially impacting IBS symptoms. When your gut bacteria are balanced, they help control bowel movements and reduce IBS symptoms like bloating. Overusing antibiotics can make them less effective in the future.

Genetics can influence microbiome dysbiosis in IBS by determining the initial composition of gut bacteria, which may predispose individuals to specific microbial imbalances. Genetic variations can impact the immune system's response to gut bacteria, contributing to dysbiosis and exacerbating IBS symptoms.

The specific mechanisms by which gut dysbiosis contributes to IBS are still being investigated. More research is required to determine the effectiveness of interventions targeting the gut microbiome for IBS treatment.

Microbiome-based therapies for IBS

Probiotics, live microorganisms found in foods like yoghurt, can help restore the equilibrium of gut bacteria. Other treatments include prebiotics and non-digestible fibres found in foods like fruits and vegetables, which promote the growth of beneficial gut bacteria.

Dietary interventions, such as a low FODMAP diet (which includes avoiding specific types of carbohydrates known to cause bloating and discomfort in certain individuals) or gluten-free diets, can help manage IBS symptoms by reducing gut inflammation and improving overall gut health. These approaches highlight the potential of targeting the gut microbiome to reduce symptoms and improve the quality of life for individuals with IBS.

Faecal microbiota transplantation (FMT) is a more invasive procedure that involves transferring faecal matter from a healthy donor to the patient's gut. It potentially restores microbial balance and has been shown to be effective in some cases.

Microbiome-based therapies are a promising area of research for managing IBS. While more research is needed, early studies suggest that these therapies may offer effective treatment options for IBS. Ongoing research on the specific microbial taxa associated with IBS is expected to provide further insights and potential treatment avenues.

Using animal models, like mice and rats, is essential for studying microbiome dysbiosis in IBS. However, these models come with limitations because they may need to fully represent the complexity of the human condition. This relatively new research area offers promising avenues for managing IBS. These therapies work by altering the composition of the gut bacteria, which is thought to play a role in developing IBS.

It is important to note that ethical considerations in microbiome-based therapies for IBS and their long-term effects are yet to be fully understood. The collection of extensive data about patients' gut microbiome and health status should be diverse and reflective of the population. This data should be shared, stored, and accessed mindfully, ensuring responsible and ethical practices in healthcare.

Simple tools such as the stool test, Bristol stool chart with bowel movements, and IBS symptoms tracker offer further understanding of microbiome imbalance for individuals with IBS, both new and long-term.

Stool test

When and where?

Stool (human faeces or poop) tests are typically performed when individuals are experiencing gastrointestinal symptoms or as part of routine health screenings. Suppose you have symptoms such as abdominal pain and alterations in bowel habits, bloating, or digestive discomfort, your healthcare provider might suggest a stool test to evaluate the status of your gut microbiome and identify any underlying issues.

Stool tests can be conducted at various healthcare facilities, including hospitals, clinics, and laboratories. Some tests may also be available for at-home collection, where individuals collect a stool sample and send it to a laboratory for analysis. Your healthcare provider can offer personalised guidance based on your symptoms and medical history to determine the ideal course of action.

Why?

Stool tests offer valuable insights into the composition and health of the gut microbiome by analysing the microbial communities present in faecal samples. These tests can provide information about the diversity and abundance of bacteria, fungi, viruses, and other microorganisms inhabiting the gut. By identifying specific microbial species and their relative proportions, stool tests can assess the overall balance of the microbiome and detect any imbalances or dysbiosis that may be associated with health conditions such as IBS.

Furthermore, stool tests can detect gut health biomarkers, such as short-chain fatty acids (SCFAs) generated by beneficial bacteria during the fermentation of dietary fibres. SCFAs are critical in maintaining gut barrier function, modulating immune responses, and regulating inflammation.

Stool tests may assess markers of gut inflammation, intestinal permeability (leaky gut), and levels of digestive enzymes and metabolites, providing comprehensive insights into gastrointestinal health.

Overall, stool tests serve as valuable tools for healthcare providers to assess the gut microbiome's composition and function. They guide personalised interventions such as dietary modifications, probiotic supplementation, and lifestyle changes, empowering individuals to manage their gut health effectively and reduce symptoms associated with conditions like IBS.

A diagnostic tool for evaluating faecal characteristics

The Bristol Stool Chart or Meyers Scale is a helpful tool for assessing bowel movements. It helps identify when to seek medical advice for issues like diarrhoea or constipation. Stools falling on extreme ends of the scale can indicate health concerns. Healthcare providers use this chart to assess bowel movements and digestive health during assessments to guide diagnoses and treatments, ensuring optimal bowel health.

Key: research suggests that it is not necessary to have a bowel movement every day. The frequency of bowel movements can vary from person to person, and it is considered normal to have anywhere from three bowel movements per week to three per day. However, a change in bowel movements in IBS-C can be a sign of:

- Constipation which is defined as having fewer than three bowel movements per week,
- Having difficulty passing stools that are hard and dry,
- Straining during bowel movements or
- Feeling like you haven't completely emptied your bowels.

My IBS-C journey involves stomach pain or cramps, which tend to worsen feeling sluggish after eating and improve after a bowel movement. These symptoms can persist for hours, days, or weeks, with the duration of a flare-up varying based on its cause and can significantly impact quality of life. A 20-minute post lunch walk reduces the feeling of sluggishness, and drinking a glass of warm water with apple cider vinegar on an empty stomach in the morning helps with bowel movements. In IBS-C, over a quarter of stools are hard or lumpy, while less than a quarter are loose or watery.

The visual aid below is used to classify stool consistency into seven categories, ranging from hard lumps (type 1) to watery diarrhoea (type 7) based on its shape and consistency, from well-formed to loose.

Goal: all individuals with IBS symptoms would aim for type 3 to type 4 stools, which indicate healthy bowel movements that are usually denser and sink in water. This sinking tendency is often associated with well-formed stools and indicates a healthy digestive system. Type 1 represents constipation, while type 7 indicates diarrhoea. Consider keeping a Bristol Stool Chart diary to track your bowel movements. This can assist you in recognising patterns or variations, providing valuable insights into your digestive health.

BRISTOL STOOL CHART		
Type 1	Separate hard lumps	Very constipated
Type 2	Lumpy and sausage like	Slightly constipated
Type 3	A sausage shape with cracks in the surface	Normal
Type 4	Like a smooth, soft sausage or snake	Normal
Type 5	Soft blobs with clear-cut edges	Lacking fibre
Type 6	Mushy consistency with ragged edges	Inflammation
Type 7	Liquid consistency with no solid pieces	Inflammation

Image by Cabot Health from Wikimedia Commons

When using the Bristol Stool Chart, it is essential to avoid the following proactive actions:

1. Overlooking changes: ignoring significant changes in stool appearance or consistency can hinder early detection of potential health issues. Stay vigilant and report any notable changes to your healthcare provider. Likewise, as you age or experience hormonal fluctuations like pregnancy or menstruation, your stool frequency and texture may be affected, which is to be expected.
2. Self-diagnosis: while the Bristol Stool Chart can provide insights into bowel health, self-diagnosing based solely on stool appearance is not advisable. Always seek advice from a healthcare professional for accurate diagnosis and treatment.
3. Neglecting other symptoms: relying solely on stool appearance may overlook other accompanying symptoms that could indicate underlying health concerns. Pay attention to additional symptoms like abdominal pain, blood in stool, or persistent changes in bowel habits.
4. Delaying medical attention: regardless of stool appearance, persistent symptoms should prompt timely medical evaluation. Delaying seeking medical attention can lead to complications or delays in treatment for underlying conditions.
5. Disregarding lifestyle factors: lifestyle factors such as diet, hydration, stress levels, environmental changes due to travel and medication use can significantly impact stool appearance. Consider how these factors affect your bowel movements and discuss any concerns with your healthcare provider.

Three steps to self-monitor your stool consistency

It may be helpful to regularly follow the three steps below to track changes in your IBS symptoms and bowel habits over time and compare them with your past self-assessments. This is a possible proactive measure before seeking professional advice. Consider using these steps to identify patterns, monitor progress, and better manage your IBS symptoms that affect stool frequency and consistency.

1. Track your IBS symptoms:
   - Choose a personalised self-tracking method: a dedicated IBS symptom tracker app, a paper journal, or a spreadsheet.
   - Record symptoms regularly: note the frequency, severity, and duration of your IBS symptoms, such as abdominal pain, bloating, gas, diarrhoea, and constipation.
   - Identify potential triggers: pay attention to what you eat, drink, and do before experiencing IBS symptoms. This could help you identify possible triggers to avoid or manage.

2. Monitor your bowel movements:
   - Use the Bristol stool chart on the previous page to help classify your stool consistency and form, providing insights into potential digestive issues.
   - Record bowel movement details and note the frequency, consistency, volume, and any other relevant observations about your bowel movements.

3. Consult your doctor for further advice:
   If your stool regularity and consistency differ from type 3 or 4, as discussed on the Bristol stool chart, consider sharing your tracking data with your doctor. They might have their own tracking tools. Your doctor can then offer personalised advice and support if your diet, lifestyle, and stress management changes are ineffective.

Based on your identified patterns and triggers, doctors might advise you on treatments like probiotics, mindfulness practices, or cognitive-behavioural therapy to manage your symptoms. This advice will vary for each person, so it is advisable to consult your doctor.

Remember: consistency is key with the above three steps. Tailor your approach following the doctor's advice because what helps one person with IBS might not help another. Symptoms change, so keep adapting as you go.

While these IBS tracker tools are valuable, it is essential to remember that they are not a substitute for professional medical advice where medical intervention is vital. Consulting a healthcare professional is necessary to diagnose, treat, and manage IBS and related dysbiosis. It is important to note that these tools may only be suitable for some. Individuals experiencing severe IBS symptoms or other underlying health conditions should consult their healthcare provider before using them.

CHAPTER RECAP:

An imbalance in gut bacteria, called dysbiosis, can contribute to the onset of IBS symptoms. A healthy microbiome supports digestion and overall well-being, while dysbiosis can cause bloating, abdominal pain, and other issues. Factors like diet, stress, genetics, and medications like antibiotics can disrupt the balance of gut bacteria. Antibiotics should only be taken if really required and prescribed by the doctor. Reducing processed sugars and stress can support a healthier microbiome. Excessive antibiotic use can also harm gut bacteria, so antibiotics should be used only when necessary.

Microbiome-based therapies aim to restore the balance of gut bacteria. These therapies include prebiotics, which are non-digestible fibres that promote the growth of beneficial bacteria; probiotics, which are live microorganisms found in foods like yoghurt that can help restore gut balance; and faecal microbiota transplantation, which involves transferring faecal matter from a healthy donor to an individual with IBS to restore microbial balance. Dietary interventions like low FODMAP and gluten-free diets can also reduce gut inflammation and improve overall health.

Stool tests analyse the gut microbiome, helping identify imbalances and guiding treatment plans. The Bristol Stool Chart assists in evaluating stool consistency and identifying possible digestive problems. Tracking bowel movements can provide insights into digestive health.

Regularly monitoring symptoms and bowel movements can help identify patterns and triggers. Tools like symptom trackers and stool charts can aid in managing IBS following the doctor's advice.

Managing IBS involves understanding your unique triggers and making informed dietary choices. While these strategies can help, consulting healthcare professionals for personalised advice and treatment is crucial.

Gluten-Free, Onion-Free & Garlic-Free Microbiome Solutions

"If you have the knowledge, let others light their candles in it." — Margaret Fuller

This chapter will discuss various dietary strategies for managing IBS, focusing on gluten-free, onion-free, and garlic-free microbiome solutions. We learned about the impact of gluten on IBS symptoms and how eliminating gluten-containing foods can reduce discomfort for some individuals. We will look into the benefits of adopting an onion and garlic-free diet, recognising these common triggers for IBS and trying alternative cooking methods. We will examine the Low FODMAP diet and its effectiveness in managing IBS symptoms by reducing the intake of fermentable carbohydrates. Finally, we will discuss the role of fibre in IBS and how incorporating soluble and insoluble fibre-rich foods can support digestive health. By learning about and applying these dietary strategies, individuals with IBS can manage their symptoms, resulting in a notable enhancement in their overall quality of life.

As an individual with IBS, including those with gluten, lactose, onion and garlic intolerance, it is essential to be mindful of these triggers when seeking relief. Here are some suggestions that may help reduce symptoms:

8. Dietary Strategies for Managing IBS

"Nothing ever becomes real till experienced." — John Keates

Dealing with IBS is not easy, but I have found that making smart food choices can really help. Here is what I have discovered:

Eat three balanced meals each day to maintain regularity. Avoid skipping meals or eating late at night, as inconsistent eating patterns can worsen symptoms. Opt for smaller meal sizes, which may help ease discomfort. Mindful eating can help reduce stress on the digestive system and improve overall digestion.

Limit alcohol consumption, aiming for at least two alcohol-free days each week. **Tip:** by eliminating alcohol intake, you may experience fewer digestive disturbances and a more regular bowel pattern, as I have observed over the past four years. Quitting alcohol entirely has made a big difference for me by reducing abdominal irritation and pain. This change has also been beneficial with age, improving digestive health and well-being.

Cut back on caffeine-containing beverages, aiming for no more than two 200 ml cups of decaffeinated versions daily or try the 3-Spice tea mix in the chapter 'quick tips for managing IBS flare-ups at home'. Decrease consumption of carbonated drinks to once a month or eliminate and prioritise hydration by drinking at least eight cups of fluids daily, focusing on drinking warm water for better bowel movement or herbal teas like peppermint tea and matcha. Staying hydrated can reduce the craving for caffeinated beverages, which is a win-win. **Try this for managing IBS:** eliminate carbonated drinks from your diet and substitute them with green tea, matcha or warm water. This approach has personally helped me achieve improved digestion.

Consume anti-inflammatory foods such as fatty fish, turmeric, and leafy greens often. These foods can help lower gut inflammation and reduce IBS symptoms.

CHAPTER RECAP:

Managing IBS through dietary strategies involves maintaining regularity in meals, avoiding triggers like alcohol and caffeine, and prioritising hydration with warm water or herbal teas. Experimenting with anti-inflammatory foods and mindful eating practices can also relieve symptoms.

Remember, everyone's experience with IBS is unique. Finding the right dietary approach may take time and patience. By listening to your body and making adjustments based on your feelings, you can discover what works for managing your symptoms effectively. Minor adjustments can significantly improve your gut health and overall well-being.

Everyone's IBS is different, so finding the proper diet might take some time. Remember to pay attention to your body and modify your diet according to how you feel. Feel free to experiment until you find what works for your body. This process of adaptation and experimentation can be empowering and motivating, as it allows you to take charge of your health and well-being.

9. Gluten-Free Diet and it's Impact on IBS

"Real difficulties can be overcome, it is only the imaginary ones that are unconquerable." — Theodore N. Vail

Cutting out gluten may help some individuals with IBS feel better. However, it is not the answer for everyone. Though IBS is not directly caused by gluten problems, some studies suggest that some with IBS feel better when they skip gluten. Here is why:
- There will be less inflammation since gluten can inflate the gut, making IBS symptoms like stomach pain, bloating, and bowel movements worse.
- Better digestion is important for those with a minor gluten intolerance; not eating it can help their stomach function better and reduce bloating pain.
- Fewer FODMAPs, where most foods with gluten, also have FODMAPs, which can mess with IBS. Skipping gluten can mean eating fewer FODMAPs, which might make symptoms better.

Going gluten-free

If you are thinking about eliminating gluten from your diet, you have to be super careful. Gluten hides in many foods, like those that are processed or have sauce or seasoning. Here is what to do:
- Check product labels carefully to spot words like wheat, barley, rye, or gluten. Hidden sources of gluten can lurk in unexpected places, such as sauces, seasonings, and even certain medications. By being diligent about ingredient labels, individuals can ensure they are genuinely eliminating gluten from their diet.
- Talk to a dietitian or doctor who knows about IBS to get tips on doing the gluten-free diet right if your personal triggers are unique.
- Try new foods such as grains without gluten, such as quinoa, millet, and rice. Also, try different fruits, vegetables, lean meats, and healthy fats to keep your meals tasty and balanced.

It is important to note that the effectiveness of a gluten-free diet for managing IBS can vary from person to person. While some individuals may experience significant improvement, others may not notice the difference. This shows that IBS is complicated, and everyone's dietary needs differ. Getting advice from a doctor or dietitian who can give you personalised help is ideal.

Going gluten-free for IBS can be a journey. It takes time and testing to see what works for you. By knowing how IBS and gluten fit together, you can make intelligent choices for your gut health. **Remember**, it is not just about gluten; it is a mix of things that can help you feel better in the long run.

CHAPTER RECAP:

While IBS is not directly triggered by gluten, some individuals with IBS find relief when they avoid it altogether. Finding what makes you feel better is a journey. It is not only about gluten but also about other factors like stress, diet, and lifestyle. Some IBS is caused by stress, while others are affected by diet and lifestyle, too.

10. Onion & Garlic-Free Diet and it's Benefits for IBS

"Never give up. No one knows what's going to happen next." — Hafez

Onion and garlic are common high triggers for various types of IBS. These foods contain high fermentable carbohydrates known as high FODMAPs, which may induce symptoms in some individuals with IBS, such as bloating and gas. Besides onion and garlic, other high FODMAP foods comprise specific fruits (such as apples and pears), certain vegetables (such as cauliflower and broccoli), and certain grains (like wheat and rye). **Tip:** if you find it challenging to pinpoint problematic foods, try eating them in isolation for a few days. While some individuals with IBS also have gluten intolerance, it is crucial to distinguish between coeliac disease (an autoimmune condition caused by gluten) and non-coeliac gluten sensitivity, which can also aggravate IBS symptoms. Individuals need to learn their own triggers through trial and error.

Bonus tip: change your cooking methods for onion and garlic or eliminate consuming them. The standard cooking methods include:
1. Infusing in oil: creating flavoured oils by infusing them with onion and garlic.
2. Stir-frying: sautéing onion and garlic in oil as a base for many dishes.
3. Roasting: cooking whole or chopped onion and garlic in the oven until caramelised and tender.
4. Boiling: adding onion and garlic to soups, stews, or broths for flavour.
5. Grilling: cook onion and garlic until charred and smoky.
6. Pickling: preserving onion and garlic in a vinegar-based solution for a tangy flavour.

These cooking methods and the form of onion and garlic can influence IBS symptoms differently. It is essential to know your triggers through trial and error. Those with IBS may eliminate onion and garlic entirely since they are high in FODMAPs. This can vary by person, so knowing your triggers through detailed trial and error is essential.

Try changing your cooking methods or cutting out onion and garlic for a few weeks to see if your symptoms improve. Monitor changes in symptoms to determine if there is a correlation. Reintroduce onion and garlic into your diet one at a time after the elimination period. Observe if symptoms return, indicating a trigger effect.

Eliminating onion and garlic, as common triggers, can reduce bloating, gas, and discomfort, making digestion more comfortable and symptoms more straightforward to manage. Personally, avoiding onion and garlic for over four years has helped me with bloating, extreme diarrhoea when specifically consuming onions, and discomfort from my IBS-C symptoms. I avoid fermenting or marinating with onion and garlic, and I exclude onion and garlic powder. This might vary for you. Explore alternative flavour enhancers such as fresh herbs, citrus zest, or mild spices to add depth to your dishes without triggering IBS discomfort.

Consider experimenting with unconventional cooking methods like marinating or fermenting, as these may affect IBS symptoms differently. Embracing creativity in your culinary journey may lead to surprising solutions that bring relief and enjoyment to your meals, all while managing your IBS symptoms effectively.

An onion and garlic-free diet can primarily help with IBS symptoms. Changing how you cook or remove them from your diet can make a big difference. Find what suits you and stick to it, as these vital base ingredients can trigger symptoms for days if not weeks. This can vary from person to person with IBS symptoms.

CHAPTER RECAP:

For some completely avoiding onion and garlic can significantly help with IBS symptoms. Experiment with different cooking methods and alternative flavour enhancers to find the preferred choice. Personally, eliminating these trigger foods has helped me manage bloating and discomfort from my IBS-C symptoms. Be creative in your culinary journey and stick to what suits you to reduce IBS symptoms over time effectively. Keep experimenting with your food, but avoid being too restrictive with your diet.

11. Low FODMAP Diet: How It Helps With IBS Symptoms

"The beginning is the most important part of the work." — Plato

FODMAP stands for Fermentable Oligosaccharides, Disaccharides, Monosaccharides, and Polyols. These are certain carbohydrates and sugar alcohols that our small intestines do not digest well. When they reach the colon, they ferment and result in bloating, gas, stomach pain, and changes in bowel habits. This is especially true for individuals with IBS or other gut problems. By eating fewer high-FODMAP foods, those with sensitive digestion can often manage their symptoms better.

A low FODMAP diet can help manage IBS and other digestive issues by avoiding certain foods. Here are some high FODMAP foods to avoid or eat in small portions, as personal triggers can vary:

- Fruits: apples, pears, watermelon, cherries, and plums.
- Vegetables: onions, garlic, and cauliflower.
- Dairy: milk, yoghurt, soft cheeses, and ice cream.
- Grains: wheat, rye, and barley.
- Legumes: beans, lentils, and chickpeas.
- Sweeteners: honey, high-fructose corn syrup, and artificial sweeteners like sorbitol and mannitol.

These restrictions can be strict but are usually temporary. Foods are gradually reintroduced to see what you can tolerate.

Many individuals with IBS find significant relief by adhering to a low FODMAP diet, which includes avoiding or limiting foods high in fermentable carbohydrates. This approach, often done under the guidance of a healthcare provider or dietician, can bring a sense of hope and optimism. In my experience, following a low FODMAP diet leads to nutrient deficiencies. Therefore, it is crucial to carefully consider your options. Getting a prompt and comprehensive annual complete body check-up to proactively detect any nutritional deficiencies is critical. I personally found out about a nutrition deficiency when I underwent mine at Apollo Hospital in Chennai, India. I have experienced firsthand thoroughness and efficiency of Apollo Hospital in Chennai, India, for an annual full-body test. I now opt for a balanced, nutritious diet that avoids the highest trigger foods and consumes the rest in moderation with an active lifestyle.

Understanding IBS and nutrient absorption

Those with IBS may face difficulties with nutrient absorption, although IBS itself typically does not directly cause malabsorption. However, prolonged symptoms such as constipation or diarrhoea in IBS can disturb the balance of gut bacteria or lead to inflammation in the intestines, potentially affecting nutrient absorption.

Research indicates that inadequate levels of Vitamin D might contribute to both IBS and mental health conditions, and it is also believed to influence central hypersensitivity. However, chronic fatigue in IBS is generally not linked to Vitamin D deficiency because many individuals without IBS may take Vitamin D supplements. Iron deficiency and anaemia are common causes of ongoing fatigue in individuals with IBS.

To address potential issues with nutrient absorption associated with IBS, it is essential to:

- Maintain a balanced diet of fibre, fruits, vegetables, and lean proteins to support overall gut health.
- Stay hydrated and active to regulate bowel movements and prevent digestive discomfort.
- Consider probiotics under medical guidance to help maintain a healthy gut flora balance.

Seeking personalised advice and management of IBS symptoms and any concerns regarding nutrient absorption from a healthcare professional is crucial. This emphasis on professional guidance can make the audience feel reassured and supported in their journey to manage their condition. For further information, reliable sources such as healthcare providers can provide additional details.

Low FODMAP diet limitations

The low FODMAP diet has gained recognition for its potential to reduce IBS systems by lowering the intake of fermentable carbohydrates in certain foods like onions, garlic, and gluten-containing grains. While many individuals with IBS have reported significant improvements in symptoms, it is essential to note that the effectiveness of this diet can vary from person to person. Individual tolerance levels, dietary preferences, and overall health may impact the effectiveness of the low FODMAP diet in relieving IBS symptoms. As such, while the diet can be a valuable tool for managing IBS, it's impact may vary between individuals.

Successfully adhering to a low FODMAP diet involves meticulous planning and careful reading of food labels, which can be challenging and time-consuming. Acknowledging the diet's challenges can make the audience feel understood and validated in their struggles. Restricting certain high FODMAP foods may lead to inadequate intake of essential nutrients such as fibre, vitamins, and minerals, potentially impacting overall health. Adhering to a strict low FODMAP diet may limit social activities involving food, leading to feelings of isolation or exclusion in social settings. The low FODMAP diet is structured with a short-term elimination phase and a reintroduction phase to identify trigger foods. However, some individuals may need help to maintain long-term wellness. Responses to the low FODMAP diet vary among individuals, and what works for one person may not work for another. Finding the right approach for each individual may take time and experimentation. Some individuals may inadvertently over-restrict their diet, eliminating too many foods unnecessarily, which can lead to inadequate nutrition and dietary limitations.

Potential solutions

For all IBS types, aim to strike a balance with a holistic approach to health by following a low FODMAP diet that avoids your extreme food triggers while still enjoying a nutritious, varied diet in moderation. This may include some high FODMAP foods that are within your tolerance limits.

In addition to the above, consider incorporating probiotics and vitamin D tablets, mainly if prescribed. These are most effectively absorbed with healthy fats such as nuts or avocado. Iron from sources like millets, specifically ragi millet, can also be beneficial. Other helpful strategies include maintaining a high-fibre diet, practising mindfulness and stress reduction techniques, eating small but frequent meals and staying well-hydrated, and checking if medium to moderate trigger foods have changed your symptoms by experimenting every 6 months or so. If natural home remedies do not provide relief, it is advisable to seek professional guidance. Persistence and a positive outlook are crucial in managing these strategies effectively.

CHAPTER RECAP:

The low FODMAP diet is known to help reduce IBS symptoms by reducing fermentable carbohydrates found in certain foods. Yet, its effectiveness varies depending on tolerance levels and overall health. Following this diet requires careful planning and label reading, which can be challenging and may result in insufficient intake of vital nutrients such as fibre, vitamins, and minerals. Strict adherence to the diet may limit social activities involving food. Maintaining it over the long term can present challenges.

Most foods contain FODMAPs, which many individuals do not digest well. Still, if you do not have IBS, you usually do not feel any digestive problems or IBS flare-ups. Only avoid FODMAPs if they make your IBS symptoms worse. They are in many foods, including healthy ones, but only prevent the big IBS triggers like onion and garlic if they are your personal worst IBS triggers. Or, if your IBS acts up, have just small amounts of medium or low-trigger foods, maybe once every three days or once a week. Experiment with your food and sometimes consume medium-trigger foods to see how your body reacts. This helps to add variety to your IBS diet only if symptoms are not troubling.

Solutions include finding a balance by incorporating some high FODMAP foods within tolerance limits, natural probiotics, a high-fibre diet, mindfulness, stress reduction, and seeking professional guidance if required, emphasising perseverance and a positive mindset.

12. Understanding How Fibre Works In IBS

"Times flies over us, but leaves its shadow behind." — Nathaniel Hawthorne

Do fibre sources, cooking methods, and the way the body operates work differently for those with IBS? Yes, fibre sources, cooking methods, and individual digestive processes can all interact differently in individuals with IBS, so let's explore this further.

Fibre is essential for maintaining digestive health. Soluble fibre is found in oats, beans, and fruits, while insoluble fibre is found in whole grains, vegetables, and nuts.

Soluble and insoluble fibre can benefit individuals with IBS, but their effects depend on the symptoms experienced. It is wise to include a variety of fibre-rich foods in your diet and observe how they affect you.

While soluble and insoluble fibre adds bulk to stool, soluble fibre is more beneficial for managing constipation and diarrhoea in IBS. In contrast, insoluble fibre primarily supports overall digestive health and bowel regularity.

Soluble fibre

- Role in IBS: soluble fibre plays a vital role by dissolving in water and forming a gel-like substance in the digestive tract. This process helps absorb water and soften stool, making bowel movements more regular and easing constipation.
- Benefit for IBS-C: adds bulk to stool and promotes regular bowel movements, relieving constipation.
- Management of diarrhoea: it can help manage diarrhoea by absorbing excess water and slowing down the digestive process, contributing to better symptom management.

Insoluble fibre

- Insoluble fibre plays a role in IBS by not dissolving in water but instead adding bulk to stool. This helps support bowel regularity by speeding up food movement through the digestive system.
- Benefit for IBS-D: while insoluble fibre may worsen symptoms for some individuals with IBS, particularly those with diarrhoea-predominant IBS (IBS-D), it can still benefit others by supporting overall digestive health and relieving constipation.
- Management of constipation: insoluble fibre promotes healthy digestion. It can help prevent constipation by facilitating the passage of waste through the intestines, contributing to better symptom management. **Personal tip:** incorporating a handful or two of fresh vegetables and salads into every meal significantly relieved my constipation.

Finding the right amount of fibre and how to do it practically

Adults should strive to consume approximately 30 grams of fibre daily. In contrast, children's fibre needs vary by ages 1 to 18, ranging from 19 to 25 grams daily. Finding the right balance between fibre types is essential based on individual symptoms and tolerances. Balancing fibre intake is vital because too much can cause bloating. At the same time, too little can worsen constipation, especially for IBS-C. **Tip:** gradually introduce fibre into your diet with at least 200 ml fluid simultaneously. With the total 30 grams adult fibre intake per day, aim to stay hydrated with at least 6-8 glasses, which is 1.5 to 2 litres of water per day for adults. This excluded alcohol and caffeinated drinks, and adding fresh lemon or lime to water helps to encourage water consumption. **Personal tip:** having a 2-litre flask or bottle with you is handy for tracking and meeting your daily water intake goals. This helps with your fibre intake and keeps your bowel movements regular. Leafy greens, root vegetables, and squash varieties are beneficial for promoting regular bowel movements in individuals with IBS-C.

Start by noticing how your tummy feels, whether it is hard to pass bowels, too much poop, or both. If you strain to poop or have both issues, try eating foods like gluten free oats, beans, and fibre rich fruits like kiwi and berries to see if it improves your bowel movements. Pay attention to how your body reacts. If it helps you have better bowel movements without causing issues, it might be suitable for you. If you frequently pass stool or desire more regular bowel movements, include foods like whole grains, vegetables, and nuts in your diet. Try to eat fibre-rich foods, and adjust your intake based on your feelings. Drinking plenty of water, especially when consuming more fibre-rich foods, can help prevent constipation. If unsure of what is good for you, consult a doctor or dietitian for personalised advice based on your symptoms.

Include a diverse range of whole plant foods such as fruits, vegetables, whole grains, starchy foods, beans, nuts, and seeds, as they are packed with fibre and beneficial for your body. Choose high-fibre foods like entire gluten-free bread, brown or overnight soaked wild rice, oats, quinoa and more. Incorporate beans and legumes like lentils and chickpeas into your diet in moderation, even if they cause gas unless you have an allergy or specific medical advice against them. Use black beans and black chickpeas in soups, salads, and meals for extra fibre. **Bonus tip:** black chickpeas are often a better choice for those with IBS because they have increased fibre content and a reduced glycemic index compared to white chickpeas. The extra fibre helps with digestion and bowel movements, while the lower glycemic index helps stabilise blood sugar levels. Some individuals find black chickpeas easier to digest, leading to less bloating and discomfort. Overall, picking black chickpeas can be a helpful choice for managing IBS symptoms.

If possible, eat fruits and vegetables with the skin on, as this is where a lot of the fibre is, like potatoes and cucumbers.

Sweet potatoes with a lower glycemic index tend to have slightly more fibre than regular potatoes, especially when consumed with the skin on. Yet having a variety of potatoes and other fibre-rich foods in moderation is vital. Pair your roasted potatoes with a creamy, high-protein lactose Greek yoghurt dip with a splash of lemon juice for added zest and chopped fresh herbs like dill or chives for more flavour that also soothes IBS for a satisfying and nutritious snack or side dish. This makes for a balanced, gut-friendly protein and fibre-rich dish that will surely please your taste buds and tummy. Experiment with your protein and fibre intake by including a range of complex carbohydrates in your diet. For example, boiled potatoes have more healthy complex carbohydrates than fried potatoes.

Personal tip: apples and pears trigger my IBS-C, so I have chosen to avoid them, while this might vary for you. Snack on nuts and seeds like overnight-soaked almonds, walnuts, and chia seeds for added fibre and nutrients. Drink plenty of water to support your digestion. Start slowly if you are not used to eating much fibre to avoid stomach issues, and gradually increase your intake over time.

Monitoring portion sizes and paying attention to individual tolerance levels is critical. Excessive consumption or specific cooking methods, such as excessive extra virgin olive oil or other oils to sauté fibre-rich foods, may increase symptoms in some individuals. They might use less oil or opt for baking or roasting with fewer hot spices, especially for those with IBS. Using the body type dosha quiz link from the chapter 'Potential Impact of Body Types on IBS' can potentially provide further insights. It is not just about the variety of fibre-rich foods; how you cook them and how often you eat them also matters.

CHAPTER RECAP:

We examined how fibre sources, cooking methods, and individual digestion vary for individuals with IBS. Fibre is essential for digestion, and there are two types: soluble and insoluble. Soluble fibre dissolves in water and helps constipation, while insoluble fibre adds bulk to stool and promotes regular bowel movements.

Finding the right balance of fibre is fundamental, as too much can cause bloating, and too little can worsen constipation. Start by noticing how your body reacts to fibre-rich foods like oats, beans, fruits, and vegetables. Make sure to drink plenty of water, especially when eating fibre-rich foods, to help with bowel movements, especially for those with IBS-C.

Experiment with cooking methods and portion sizes to find what works. If symptoms worsen, avoid IBS triggers like apples and pears, and snack on nuts and seeds for added fibre. Pay attention to your body's response and adjust accordingly. **Remember**, not just what you eat but how you cook and eat that matters in managing IBS symptoms.

Optimising Your Microbiome

"If you want to make life easy, make it hard." — Johann Wolfgang von Goethe

This chapter will discuss how to keep your gut bacteria healthy. We will focus on three main areas: understanding the importance of good bacteria and the foods that support them, exploring lifestyle habits that benefit your gut, and identifying the optimal foods for gut health.

Optimising your gut microbiome refers to promoting a healthy balance of gut microorganisms, known as the microbiome, through various lifestyle and dietary strategies. This includes the below approaches. The goal is to support overall gut health and enhance digestion, sustained immunity, and well-being.

13. Probiotics and Prebiotics: Their Role In Gut Health

"The best way to predict the future is to create it." — Abraham Lincoln

A gut feeling

Our gut is home to trillions of microorganisms, collectively known as the gut microbiota. This complex ecosystem plays a crucial role in our overall health, influencing digestion, immunity, and even mental well-being.

Probiotics and prebiotics are two key players in maintaining a healthy gut. Let's explore their roles and potential benefits for managing IBS symptoms. Probiotics are live bacteria found in fermented food like yoghurt and kimchi that have live and active cultures which are beneficial for your digestive system, while prebiotics are types of non-digestible fibres found in fruits, vegetables, and whole grains or added to yoghurt and breakfast cereals that serve as food for these beneficial bacteria. While some bad bacteria may also utilise prebiotics, the main function or prebiotics is to support the growth and activity of good bacteria, thereby promoting a healthy gut microbiome.

Studies suggest that specific probiotic strains like Lactobacillus Plantarum and Bifidobacterium Breve could reduce IBS-C symptoms like bloating and abdominal pain. By consuming prebiotic-rich foods, we provide nourishment to the good bacteria in our gut, allowing them to thrive and flourish. These bacteria produce short-chain fatty acids and other metabolites that contribute to gut health, enhance intestinal barrier function, and help regulate immune responses and control inflammation.

Some prefer prebiotics over probiotics. By feeding your existing probiotics, you foster the growth of good bacteria already present in your gut instead of introducing new bacteria from external sources like cows. Prebiotics help establish a stable, healthy gut microbiome, reducing the need to introduce new bacteria.

How probiotics and prebiotics may help manage IBS

A healthy balance of gut bacteria is essential for effective digestion and nutrient absorption. Both probiotics and prebiotics can help achieve this balance, reducing symptoms like bloating and gas in IBS. Probiotic strains such as Lactobacillus and Bifidobacterium possess anti-inflammatory properties, which may soothe the gut lining and reduce IBS-related pain. Probiotics and prebiotics promote regular bowel movements and improve stool consistency, potentially easing constipation in IBS.

A robust gut microbiota supports immune function, and probiotics and prebiotics can bolster immunity, lowering the risk of infections that can worsen IBS symptoms.

It is imperative to note that the effectiveness of probiotics and prebiotics for IBS varies among individuals and specific strains. Consulting a healthcare professional is advisable. Alongside probiotics and prebiotics, a fibre-rich diet and fermented foods can enhance gut health and IBS management. While research shows promise, more studies are required to fully grasp the long-term effects and optimal usage of probiotics and prebiotics for IBS.

In conclusion, probiotics and prebiotics offer potential benefits for gut health and IBS symptom relief. However, personalised guidance from a healthcare provider is essential for tailored treatment. **Personal**

tip: I intentionally avoided probiotic supplements and flavoured yoghurts and opted for natural foods like kimchi and unflavoured, unsweetened natural yoghurt with probiotic strains instead.

Incorporating fermented foods for gut health

Fermentation is a natural process where bacteria and yeast break down sugars in foods, creating beneficial compounds like probiotics that are good for gut health. Common fermented foods include yoghurt, kimchi, sauerkraut, and kombucha.

To ferment foods at home, you create the conditions for good bacteria to grow. This often involves adding salt or a starter culture and letting the food sit at room temperature. The time it takes to ferment foods at room temperature can vary a lot. It might be just a few days, or it could be a few weeks. Follow the instructions in your recipe or guide to know when it is ready.

For example, sauerkraut and kombucha usually take one to two weeks to ferment. In contrast, kimchi can take just three or five days. While fermenting, you might notice changes in how it tastes, feels, and smells.

Once your fermented food is ready and tastes just the way you like it, you can enjoy it in moderation as a side dish at least once a day. The sense of accomplishment from creating your own healthy, homemade fermented foods can be a great motivator to continue this practice. To keep it fresh, you can put it in the fridge, which slows down the fermentation. Then, you can enjoy your homemade fermented foods as a yummy and healthy part of your meals.

There are two main types of fermentation aerobic and anaerobic. Aerobic fermentation needs oxygen and is common in foods like sourdough bread. Anaerobic fermentation happens without oxygen and is found in foods like sauerkraut and kimchi.

Both types of fermentation can make tasty and healthy foods. It is just a matter of which method works well for fermenting your food. Just make sure to use clean equipment, fresh ingredients, and the right amount of salt, as too much can make your food too salty. Fermentation is a simple and natural way to preserve food to boost flavour and promote gut health. **Tip:** for individuals with IBS, there are some things to remember. Avoid fermenting certain foods that might make symptoms worse, like beans or dairy, if you are lactose (the sugar found in dairy) intolerant. Also, be cautious with highly acidic foods like citrus fruits, vinegar-based products that irritate your digestive system, and artificial sweeteners that can ferment in the gut and cause digestive issues, particularly for those with IBS. It is all about finding what works for you and your gut.

While fermenting foods, it is important to maintain the right temperature to ensure the growth of good bacteria. If the temperature is too high or too low, harmful bacteria might grow instead of good ones. Mould can grow on fermented foods, especially if not stored or exposed to air. However, with the right precautions, fermentation is a safe and natural way to preserve food. If you notice any signs like a strange smell, weird colour, or mould, it is safest to throw the food away to avoid getting sick and just make a new batch. Pay attention to too much salt and exceptionally high spice levels if you have IBS as it can cause bloating and stomach acidity along with stomach irritation.

Adding fermented foods to your diet for a healthier gut depends on what you like and how well you tolerate them. It is good to start with small amounts, like a few spoonfuls a few times a week. Then, as your body gets used to them, you can have them more often. Pay attention to how your body feels and change how much you eat based on that. **Personal tip:** watch out for high sugar in probiotic supplements like flavoured yoghurts and drinks. As a person with IBS-C, I have also avoided taking anti-bloating or anti-gas tablets for over 25 years and limited added sugar to less than one teaspoon per day by having moderate amounts of dark chocolate instead, which accelerated my results with naturally fermented foods. It is recommended to consume natural fermented foods daily for at least 4 weeks, avoid supplements to assess symptom improvement, and continue daily with natural options such as kimchi and unflavoured yoghurts. Take some time to review your food and symptom diaries, as well as your lifestyle choices, to better understand how fermented foods impact your gut health and overall well-being.

Microbiome-friendly foods

Fungicides and pesticide chemicals sprayed on crops to keep them healthy can affect our body's hormones and potentially disrupt the gut microbiome, which may impact individuals, particularly those with IBS. These chemicals make digestion and overall well-being even trickier, especially if their gut is sensitive. Residues from these chemicals on fruits and vegetables could make IBS symptoms worse. Some might notice that eating foods treated with these chemicals triggers or worsens their symptoms. Therefore, consider switching to organic produce. I have included further tips below to empower you and reduce your exposure to pesticides.

Based on recent information from the U.S. Department of Agriculture (USDA) data, you can opt for organic options from the 'dirty dozen,' as seen below, where pesticide levels are lower. Then, if you prefer, you can choose less expensive conventionally grown produce from the 'Clean Fifteen'.

The Dirty Dozen 2024 highlights a compilation of fruits and vegetables containing the highest pesticide residue provided by the Environmental Working Group, a U.S. non-profit organisation. These foods often have a large surface area and are grown in regions where pesticides are heavily used or are challenging to wash thoroughly.

1. Strawberries
2. Spinach
3. Kale, Collard and Mustard Greens
4. Grapes
5. Peaches
6. Pears
7. Nectarines
8. Apples
9. Bell & Hot Peppers
10. Cherries
11. Celery
12. Tomatoes

The Clean Fifteen 2024 are fruits and vegetables with the most minor pesticide residue. Avocados and sweet corn are at the top of the list for being the cleanest because they have thicker skins that protect them from pesticides.

1. Avocados
2. Sweet corn
3. Carrots
4. Sweet Potatoes
5. Mangoes
6. Mushrooms
7. Watermelon
8. Cabbage
9. Kiwi
10. Honeydew Melon
11. Asparagus
12. Sweet Peas (frozen)
13. Papaya
14. Onions
15. Pineapple

The USDA tested baby foods finding fewer pesticides in non-organic options than in whole fruits and vegetables, but still detected residues in 38% of products. Studies link pesticides to health issues, prompting concerns about children's safety. The EPA's handling of children's pesticide exposure is under scrutiny, urging caution and awareness, as the American Academy of Pediatrics advises.

Here are some ways to reduce pesticides in your food:

- Cleaning fruits and vegetables before eating can help reduce pesticide levels, although no washing method can completely eliminate all residues. Start by washing your hands thoroughly.
- Use running water. Wash and rub produce under running water and then soak it in white vinegar or turmeric to remove the most pesticide residue. Vinegar and turmeric might help lower pesticide levels in fruits and vegetables. But **remember**, the wise way to stay safe is by washing your produce really well before eating. That is the most important thing to do to reduce pesticide exposure.
- Avoid soap, detergent, commercial soaks or scrubs. Stick to water alone. Using a brush or scrubbing pad can also help remove surface pesticides.

- After rinsing, dry the produce with a clean cloth or paper towel. This can further reduce chemicals and bacteria that may be present on the food surface.

Try this instead: to check for artificial colours and pesticides on produce like watermelon from the "Clean Fifteen," lightly rub a tissue on the surface. If you notice an unusual colour tint on the tissue, it could indicate the presence of artificial colours or pesticides. The same applies when washing frozen blueberries or strawberries; an excessive colour bleed might suggest artificial colours or pesticide residues.

Considering the above information, the table below offers a selection of foods from diverse cultures that support a healthy gut microbiome and may help reduce IBS symptoms.

Food	Recipe
Yoghurt	Plain Greek yoghurt topped with berries and nuts
Kefir	Smoothie with kefir, banana and spinach
Fermented vegetables	Homemade sauerkraut or kimchi as a side dish
Whole grains	Quinoa, millets or brown rice grain bowls with vegetables
Beans and legumes	Lentil soup or bean chili loaded with vegetables
Fruits and vegetables	Raw carrots, bell peppers, and cucumber with hummus
Nuts and seeds	Chia or ground flaxseeds over gluten-free oatmeal or yoghurt
Miso soup	Traditional Japanese miso soup with tofu and seaweed
Tofu stir-fry	Stir-fry tofu with mixed vegetables and ginger
Kimchi fried rice	Korean-inspired fried rice with kimchi and vegetables
Lentil dal	Indian lentil dal seasoned with turmeric and cumin
Greek salad	Greek salad with cucumber, tomato olives, and feta cheese
Hummus wrap	Gluten-free wrap filled with hummus, vegetables, and falafel
Salsa verde chicken	Mexican-inspired salsa verde chicken with roasted vegetables
Coconut curry	Thai coconut curry with vegetables and tofu or chicken

Self-created table by Jan Nallathamby content from National Center for Biotechnology Information

CHAPTER RECAP:

This chapter explored how to keep your gut healthy to ease IBS symptoms using probiotics and prebiotics. These tiny organisms in our gut play a significant role in our health. Probiotics are good bacteria found in foods like yoghurt and kimchi. At the same time, prebiotics are fibres found in fruits and vegetables that feed these good bacteria. Eating these foods helps our gut bacteria grow and produce helpful substances that keep our gut healthy and reduce inflammation. Probiotics and prebiotics can aid in managing symptoms of IBS, such as bloating and constipation, by promoting a balanced gut microbiota and supporting immune function.

Fermented foods like yoghurt and sauerkraut are natural sources of probiotics that we can easily include in our daily diets. The key is to include fermented foods daily in the diet and have a portion of vegetables and salad in every meal. It is essential to choose organic produce when consuming the 'dirty dozen' fruits and vegetables whenever possible to avoid harmful pesticides that can disrupt our gut microbiome and worsen IBS symptoms. Following these tips and including microbiome-friendly foods in our diets can support our gut health and manage IBS more effectively.

14. Lifestyle Practices to Promote a Healthy Microbiome

"Good friends, good books, and a sleepy conscience: this is the ideal life." — Mark Twain

Alongside the 'dirty dozen' and 'clean fifteen' foods discussed in the previous chapter, avoiding unnecessary antibiotics to protect your gut bacteria is essential. Only use them when necessary to maintain a healthy and diverse gut microbiome. Below are more factors to consider for a healthy microbiome:

A balanced and disciplined approach with a positive mindset is essential for managing IBS	
Action Item	**How**
Reduce stress as it can hurt your gut	Meditation, yoga, or deep breathing, practised daily for 10 minutes after waking up. Engage in intentional play at all ages with all ages across all cultures if you can
Adequate sleep is good for your gut and your health	Try sleeping 7 hours daily from 10 p.m. to 5 a.m. or 9 p.m. to 4 a.m. Likewise, based on your lifestyle, flex it and follow the same sleep routine
Regular exercise is good for your overall health and gut bacteria	Stay active; and move your body every two hours the least
Hydration is essential for a healthy balance of gut bacteria and digestion	Drink at least 2 litres of filtered, clean, warm water daily
Limit sugar and processed foods. It can harm your gut bacteria	Reducing your sugar intake will reduce your sugar cravings. Within a few weeks, your taste receptors will adjust. As you start eating healthier, you will find that junk food no longer appeals to you. Choose nutritious foods, and you will begin to crave them instead.

Self-created table by Jan Nallathamby content from National Center for Biotechnology Information

Bonus tips:
- Speak to lived experts with similar IBS symptoms, then research, refine and use your judgment before action, and seek medical advice where required.
- Choose natural remedies over medications whenever possible, and consider medication only if natural options do not work. While medicines can provide quick relief, they can impact the natural gut healing process.
- Aim for long-term microbiome health by tackling your digestion issues with natural foods as much as possible.

Portion control made easy with your and ideal plate arrangement

As food has evolved with modern times, our lifestyles have shifted, often requiring less physical labour. While expending less energy via physical labour as our societal roles shift, this change impacts our dietary needs, as we may consume more processed foods and fewer fresh, whole foods. To adapt, we must prioritise nutrient-rich options and incorporate movement into our daily routines to maintain health and vitality despite reduced physical activity.

Your daily routine, how active you are, and what you want to achieve with your health all affect how much you should eat. If you are not very active, stick to meals about the size of your fist. This approach can help with managing IBS and reducing its symptoms like indigestion and bloating due to overeating. Fist-sized portions offer a straightforward way to regulate food intake, ensuring appropriate portions of protein, vegetables, carbohydrates and low-sugar fruits high in fibre. This approach prevents overeating, promotes a balanced diet, and supports digestive health, all essential for reducing IBS symptoms like bloating and constipation.

The British Heart Foundation recommends a simple method for each type of food that should be portioned separately according to the guidelines below: using your palm. For protein, aim for a portion about the size of your palm. Have two palmfuls of various coloured fresh vegetables, and carbohydrates like rice or millet should be roughly the size of your clenched fist. Balance your carbohydrate intake evenly throughout the day across each meal, and exercise daily for a healthier gut. It is essential to balance your diet for a healthy gut.

Use your palm to gauge portion sizes like protein, vegetables, fruits, fats and carbohydrates

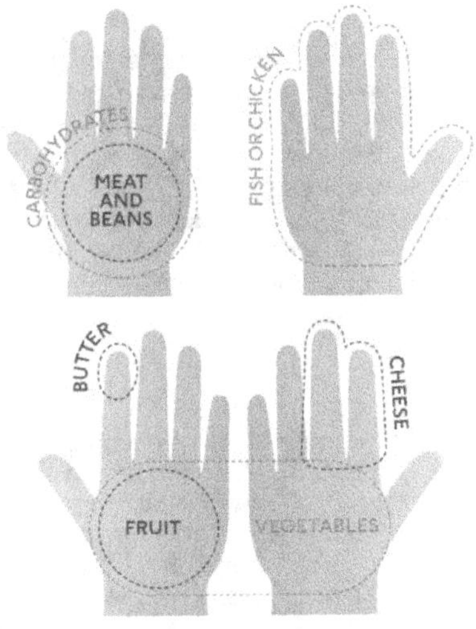

Image by British Heart Foundation 'How to get portion sizes right'

Start by eating vegetables, protein, and then carbohydrates on your plate to Optimise energy levels. This arrangement ensures you fuel your body with suitable energy sources. Research suggests that consuming carbohydrates, like whole grains, provides brain fuel, keeping your mind sharp and clear when glucose levels are consistent in each meal. Fill half your plate with vegetables, then add protein and carbohydrates to implement this. This simple adjustment can enhance energy levels and cognitive and digestive function throughout the day. **Tip:** steer clear of sugary, carbonated or alcoholic drinks with your meals, which often pack in lots of calories but offer little nutritional value. Instead, opt for warm water instead of cold water to promote a healthy and diverse gut microbiome, essential for digestion and overall well-being. Aim for two alcohol-free days a week and ideally eliminate them to help with the long-term health of your microbiome. **Recap:** remember, the amount of butter and cheese you should have is tiny. The cheese portion is about the size of one or two fingers or one small matchbox.

A smaller 9-inch diameter plate can help you eat less food overall. To stay healthy and energised, include vegetarian and non-vegetarian meals in your weekly diet based on your preferences. UK dietary guidelines recommend meat up to 3 times a week for a balanced diet. **Personal tip:** eating vegetarian meals three days each week can simplify meal planning and reduce waste by keeping vegetables fresh. This dietary choice often leaves individuals feeling lighter compared to consuming meat. For those with IBS-C, focusing on vegetables high in soluble fibre can be beneficial as they help regulate bowel movements by reducing the intake of vegetables high in insoluble fibre.

How:
- Before eating, express gratitude for your meal by saying, "Thank you for this nourishing food; may it bring joy and wellness to my day."
- Sit down to focus on your meal,
- Avoid distractions like gadgets and TV, which can lead to overeating,
- Eat slowly,
- Chewing your food thoroughly is vital for those with IBS to enable easier nutrient absorption and
- Eating about 80% complete helps digestion, especially for those with IBS. Your brain needs about 20 minutes to recognise that your stomach is full. Only eat when you feel comfortably satisfied, not overly full. Drinking a glass of water before and during meals can help you feel full and avoid overeating.

The above small, consistent daily acts can help with IBS symptom management, such as indigestion that could lead to bloating.

When:
- Space meals and never skip as it leads to overeating later in the day,
- Eating small portions 3-5 times per day is ideal to help minimise IBS symptoms and
- Pay attention to your hunger signals, and stop eating when you feel about 80% full.

Tip: those with IBS must avoid late-night eating and finish their last meal by 6 p.m. before sunset. This can benefit gut health by allowing the body more time to digest food before resting. This practice aligns with the body's natural rhythms, promoting better digestion and quality sleep.

Research suggests that late-night eating can disrupt circadian rhythms, our body's natural daily sleep-wake cycle clock. It can also interfere with digestion, potentially leading to digestive discomfort and weight gain.

Intermittent fasting for gut health

Intermittent fasting means alternating between periods of eating and fasting. It can help manage IBS by giving your digestive system time to rest and reset, and research has indicated that it can also prevent future diseases. For those with IBS, start with shorter fasting windows of 12 hours and gradually increase the duration to a maximum of 24 hours. Seek advice from a healthcare provider before starting, especially if you have any medical conditions.

Personal tip: if you are trying intermittent fasting once a week, stick with it long-term if it is safe for you, and drink warm liquids all day with one meal before sunset. For the past two years of intermittent fasting, this has helped me feel less bloated, less gas, and more relaxed and focused.

Ingredient label reading

Before trying new foods or drinks, research, taste them, and constantly review the ingredient list to prevent adverse reactions. The fewer and simpler ingredients, the better. If you note complicated names, avoid them and opt for natural, fresh whole food choices on the ingredient list. The first 2-3 ingredients are essential because they set the tone for the entire product. They are like the leading players in a recipe, affecting how it tastes, feels, and what nutrients it provides. The last ingredient contributes to the least.

If onion or garlic is listed at the end of the ingredients, it may be tolerated well in small portions. So, it is wise to check these out first and make sure they match what you are looking for regarding the position of the IBS trigger food in the ingredient food list and quality for overall daily nutrition. Ideally, you should cook at home more often. This will give you much more control over the ingredients in your food.

Dietary monotony: a holistic approach for managing IBS

The Mediterranean diet is packed with fibre-rich foods like fruits and vegetables, which promote healthy digestion and prevent constipation, a common IBS-C symptom. Healthy fats from olive oil reduce inflammation in the gut. At the same time, the diet's emphasis on whole grains provides sustained energy without aggravating digestive issues.

Incorporate lean proteins like fish and poultry, and limit red meat and processed foods. Enjoy meals mindfully, aiming for balance and variety.

Moderating oil intake and opting for less spicy, grilled foods can be beneficial for managing IBS symptoms. Try sparingly using all oils, including olive oil, especially if you have a primarily inactive lifestyle, and choosing grilled options over fried. Enjoying meals this way may help reduce discomfort and promote better digestion.

Trying different cuisine types can help IBS by providing various ingredients and cooking methods. For example, Asian cuisines often use ginger and turmeric, which have anti-inflammatory properties that can soothe the digestive system. Mediterranean cuisines emphasise olive oil and fish, which are beneficial for gut health. Exploring diverse cuisines can introduce new flavours and nutrients, reducing the risk of dietary monotony and potentially easing IBS symptoms.

Spice up your health: the benefits of sea salt and seaweed extract for IBS

Using sea salt or ground sea salt instead of regular table salt can provide essential trace minerals beneficial for gut health, especially for those with IBS. Sea salt contains minerals like magnesium, potassium, and calcium, which can support digestion and help maintain electrolyte balance.

Seaweed can help with IBS because it contains soluble fibre, which can ease constipation and regulate bowel movements. It is also rich in nutrients like iodine, calcium, iron, and antioxidants that support gut health and reduce inflammation. Seaweed adds natural flavour and nutrients without synthetic ingredients, making it a healthier option for seasoning meals. These alternatives enhance taste and contribute to better gut function, making them ideal choices for individuals managing IBS symptoms.

Liquid seaweed extract is a concentrated liquid often used in soups, sauces, and marinades for added flavour. Powdered seaweed extract, on the other hand, can be sprinkled onto dishes like salads and stir-fries to enhance their taste and nutritional value. Seaweed seasoning blends and condiments, like seaweed flakes or furikake, contain seaweed extract and other ingredients like sesame seeds, bonito flakes, or spices, adding umami flavour and texture to meals. Start with small portions and see how you feel.

Hydration hero: coconut water and water for IBS relief

Fresh coconut water is rich in electrolytes such as potassium and magnesium, which can be soothing for IBS symptoms like diarrhoea by replenishing lost fluids and minerals. Aim for one to two 250 to 500 ml servings daily, regardless of IBS type, to stay hydrated without overloading your system. Spread them out over the day for optimal hydration and electrolyte balance. However, avoid varieties with added sugars or artificial flavours, as these can worsen IBS symptoms. Opt for natural, unsweetened coconut water to manage IBS discomfort. **Personal tip:** drinking coconut water with chia seeds pre-soaked for 2 hours is a simple and nutritious way to boost hydration and add fibre to your diet. You can easily include these into your daily routine by preparing a batch of chia seeds soaked in coconut water overnight and keeping it in the fridge. Enjoy it as a refreshing drink on its own or with daily snacks like yoghurt, fruit salads, or smoothie bowls for an extra nutritional boost. It is a convenient and tasty way to stay hydrated and satisfied throughout the day while staying within your recommended calories intake per day.

Drinking warm water over cold helps maintain gut health by aiding digestion and promoting bowel movement. Cold water can shock the digestive system, while warm water soothes and helps food break down quickly. Opting for warm water supports a healthy microbiome and reduces IBS symptoms.

Warm water for gut health

Drinking 6-8 glasses (200 ml per glass) of warm water daily can help manage IBS. Staying hydrated keeps your digestive system working well, reducing constipation and bloating. Warm water relaxes your gut muscles, easing discomfort and aiding digestion by stimulating your organs and promoting smooth bowel movements. It also helps break down food more efficiently, allowing your body to absorb nutrients better. Studies show that drinking warm water can increase blood flow to the intestines and improve gut movement, reducing the risk of constipation and bloating.

To include warm water in your daily routine, replace cold drinks with warm water, especially before and after meals. Sipping warm water throughout the day helps keep you hydrated and supports digestive function. This simple change can promote a healthy microbiome and improve digestive health.

Adequate water intake softens stools, making them easier to pass, essential for those with IBS-C. **Bonus tip:** adding a slice of lemon to your warm water can enhance digestion and add a refreshing taste. Listening to your body and drinking water throughout the day can support overall gut health and improve your comfort and well-being.

Enzyme supplements

Digestive enzyme supplements are expected to assist in breaking down nutrients, especially FODMAPs, easing IBS symptoms. Avoid relying solely on digestive enzyme supplements as they might not address the root cause of digestive issues and can be expensive. Instead, natural enzyme sources like pineapple and papaya should be prioritised in meals. You should reserve enzyme supplements for occasional use when natural options have not helped, opt for supplements tailored to FODMAP digestion and seek advice from a healthcare professional for specific digestive challenges. **Tip:** experiment with natural foods and avoid supplements and drugs unless absolutely required and prescribed by a doctor, as they can unnecessarily confuse the already dysfunctional gut.

Craving crunch: managing crispy food for a happy gut

Ever wondered why we crave crispy snacks? Craving crunchy food is often tied to our feelings and thoughts. The satisfying crunch gives us a quick mood boost, especially when stressed or bored. To manage these cravings, it is essential to understand what triggers them. Stay mindful of your emotions and find healthier ways to cope, like taking a walk, distracting your mind or practising deep breathing. Keep crunchy snacks out of sight and choose more nutritious options to satisfy your craving without harming your health. You may have healthy, crunchy options such as kale or baked plantain chips, rice cakes, bell pepper strips or roasted chickpeas.

Another reason we crave crispiness is that our taste buds enjoy the contrast of textures, which is a mental note that food is fresh. However, too much crispy food can upset your stomach, especially for those with IBS. **Tip:** the key is to aim for balance in each meal. By adding crunchy nuts, while being mindful of salt content, as toppings on softer proteins and grains, you can enjoy the texture without overdoing it. Accept your cravings but manage them with a plan. Keep crispy snacks for special treats, and practice portion control. You can enjoy a happy gut without sacrificing flavour with discipline and smart choices.

Managing energy and sleep for IBS amid stress

During stressful times, managing energy levels and sleep is fundamental for individuals with IBS. Stress can worsen symptoms, leading to fatigue and disrupted sleep patterns. To cope better, prioritise relaxation techniques like deep breathing, meditation, or gentle yoga before bedtime to promote better sleep. Establish a consistent bedtime schedule and cultivate a calming bedtime routine. Avoid consuming caffeine and using screens close to bedtime, and instead, choose calming activities such as reading or taking warm baths. Regular exercise and a balanced diet help regulate energy levels and enhance sleep quality.

Smart eating strategies for IBS while travelling, at work or dining out

When dining at hotels, you could ask the chef to wash salad ingredients well to remove pesticide residue. Sharing meals can help control portion sizes, and planning takeaways in advance prevents overeating, especially with desserts and dishes like Biryani. Biryani is a dish known for its richness and spices, which can be high in fats and may not be suitable for those with IBS when consumed in large portions due to potential triggers. This approach supports healthier fat and sugar levels, reducing the risk of metabolic problems. Beware of excessive salt and sugar in packaged foods and juices. When dining out, choose dishes with natural sweetness or request alternatives to refined sugar. Balancing meals with fresh, unprocessed options such as a simple banana or other fruits low in sugar and high in fibre that you can carry from home helps effectively manage IBS symptoms like constipation.

Opt for warm water for gut health that promotes bowel movement for IBS-C. Swap alcohol and cocktails for mocktails with non-carbonated drinks or fresh, natural juices with no added sugar. Letting the waiter know your IBS dietary requirements can help them offer tailored menu choices.

Personal tip: if you can, try eating healthy proteins and fibre with lots of water at home before heading out. That way, you will have better control over your appetite and can be careful with gut-sensitive choices like alcohol and processed foods. Prioritise variety in fresh vegetable intake when eating out to aid digestion and avoid constipation. Pack travel-friendly foods for IBS relief, like salads and homemade snacks, to avoid discomfort.

Many restaurant dishes contain onions and garlic in their pre-made bases, pates, soups, stews, sauces, or marinades, which are common triggers for IBS symptoms. What is critical here is knowing your own intolerances. For example, if you find cooked garlic tricky to tolerate but can handle fresh, request a substitution in the kitchen or request to remove it altogether if both will cause problems.

Flavourings often include onion or garlic and are unsuitable for most with IBS. **Key takeaway:** just because something is labelled "gluten-free" does not necessarily mean it is IBS-friendly. Many flavourings and sauces used in gluten-free menus contain onion and garlic, which can trigger IBS symptoms for days or even weeks. Also, check if a gluten-free pie contains leeks or other ingredients that cause IBS flare-ups based on your individual intolerances.

Choose menu options without a sauce, such as grills, sushi, sashimi, stir fry, or risotto. Ask the restaurant to serve the sauce or gravy on the side in a separate dish if they cannot substitute it with a gluten-free sauce. Scrape off the gluten batter, sauce or coating from the food where possible. Check that the pizza base is gluten-free and the tomato sauce is onion- and garlic-free with less salt to avoid bloating. Use apps to find eat-outs that offer gluten-free options and provide feedback to other restaurants and cafes, encouraging them to be more IBS-friendly since it is now becoming a worldwide common dietary requirement.

Call the restaurant ahead to pre-order by asking questions about the food and if they can remove or adjust your IBS trigger ingredients. Check the online menu beforehand or ask if you can bring your homemade meal if the restaurant needs more suitable options. Planning ahead can help you avoid paying extra charges for bringing your own meal to busy restaurants. Don't hesitate to provide feedback to restaurants and social event organisers at work and friends circle to improve catering for those with IBS, onion and garlic intolerance where they can. The more individuals know, the better it is. This proactive approach ensures you enjoy social gatherings without compromising your health and social life, making you feel empowered and in control.

When dining out or travelling, it is crucial to research and plan ahead to ensure you have suitable choices available, especially if you have intolerances like onion, garlic, lactose, and gluten. Packing cumin seeds and green tea bags for digestion and bowel regularity can be a simple yet effective strategy. By requesting a hot water top-up and steeping the cumin seeds for 10 minutes, you can aid digestion. Planning ahead and being prepared can help you avoid discomfort and enjoy your dining experience.

Be bold about carrying your sauces in small bottles when dining out, at work or travelling. IBS bloating and discomfort can last for days or weeks, so it is good to have safe options when dining out or travelling.

Keep gluten-free bread, rice, corn, oat cakes, fresh salads, ground flax seed powder, fermented food, and likewise at work to accompany your balanced meals. This is helpful if you need clarification on takeout options near your workplace.

Pack a meal for dinner if you are out and need clarification on the return time. Rather than opt for mint or chewing gum after eating out, suck on 1-2 fresh cloves or uncoated fresh cumin seeds. When dealing with IBS sensitivities and cultivating a healthy gut microbiome, the more natural, the better.

Oil pulling for gut health

We all know that digestion starts in our mouth. When we eat, our tongues detect the nutrients and signal our digestive system. If our mouth is not clean, our tongue can't signal properly. Then, when food reaches our stomach, it may not be broken down well, and we might not absorb all the nutrients.

Oil pulling, an ancient Indian practice, entails swishing oil in your mouth to enhance oral health and potentially support overall well-being, including gut health. Coconut or sesame oil, provided you are not allergic to these ingredients, is often used for oil pulling. It can help remove harmful mouth bacteria, reduce overall gut bacterial load, and inhibit microbes linked to digestive issues.

Swirl a tablespoon of oil around in your mouth for 10-20 minutes while reading or listening to a podcast, and then spit the oil into a trash bin to prevent sink clogging. Include oil pulling at least twice a week, ideally daily or alternate days, right after brushing teeth and tongue cleaning and a glass of warm water, followed by a quick brisk 20-minute walk and then breakfast. Some studies suggest that oil pulling may support a healthy microbiome, improve beneficial bacteria, and improve oral health. More research is required to fully understand its impact on gut bacteria, but the potential benefits are promising.

Coconut oil is considered the best because it is safe to consume and has anti-inflammatory, antibacterial, and antimicrobial properties. However, it is important to note that oil pulling may not be suitable for everyone, and some people may experience side effects such as nausea or upset stomach. Our mouths harbour various bacteria, some beneficial and others harmful. Unlike mouthwash, oil pulling targets only harmful bacteria, which can remove helpful and harmful bacteria.

Simple habits for gut health

Staying active, eating well, and connecting with others are not only beneficial but essential to managing IBS. Stick to a routine, but add variety. These straightforward habits can empower you to take control of your IBS symptoms.

Keep an open mind to trying new habits that promote a healthy gut. Challenge yourself to explore different approaches to support your gut health. Stay curious and keep learning; finding what works for you is crucial to maintaining a healthy microbiome.

Limit or eliminate consumption of rich or fatty foods, including chips, fast food, fried food, creamy, fatty, salty sauces and sweets. Cut down on caffeine, diluted cordial, and squash drinks; opt for non-caffeinated or herbal teas instead. Watch out for added sugar, carbohydrates, and artificial flavours. Opt for natural alternatives by checking ingredients for a simple mix of 2-3 items. Control portion sizes of fresh fruits with no more than three portions of 80g per day.

Reduce screen time and delegate or outsource time-consuming tasks to reduce stress. These simple habits help control IBS symptoms and improve overall well-being.

Instead of constantly worrying about food due to IBS triggers, plan ahead and stay positive. Shift your focus from food intolerance to daily activities and creating positive experiences. For travellers with IBS, pack essentials like water, snacks, digestive aids like cumin seeds, and medications if absolutely required to manage symptoms on the go. You can enjoy your travels without letting IBS hold you back by staying prepared and maintaining a positive mindset.

Remember to sip on warm water throughout the day. Warm water can help relax the muscles of the intestines, potentially easing symptoms of IBS. It also supports digestion and aids in preventing constipation, which are common issues for people with IBS.

Lifestyle boost: fun, community, and positive vibes for IBS relief

Not only triggers and balanced food awareness, but it also surrounds you with positivity and engages in enjoyable activities that can help reduce IBS symptoms and enhance your overall well-being by promoting a healthy microbiome.

Join creative game groups or communities, spend time with positive individuals, and continue playing games regularly, regardless of age. Find local or online groups, schedule regular hangouts, and explore new hobbies. **Personal tip:** include creative game groups and communities in your daily routine to consistently enjoy their positive effects on IBS symptoms. This could include activities like board games, puzzles, or even online gaming communities.

The research underscores the pivotal role of social support and engaging activities in enhancing mental and physical health, particularly in managing chronic conditions like IBS. Regular participation in enjoyable activities and maintaining a positive social circle can lead to reduced stress levels and improved mood, thereby contributing to better health.

Navigating IBS while dating

Dating with IBS can pose challenges, from managing symptoms to feeling self-conscious about dietary restrictions. Communicate openly with your partner regarding your condition and what you require. Choose date venues with IBS-friendly options, like cafes with fresh IBS friendly meals. Prioritise activities unrelated to food, such as hiking or playing creative fun games, to keep IBS from hindering your confidence or connection.

When dating with food intolerances like IBS, open communication is vital. It is critical to consider all factors that support you in the long term, such as a helpful, flexible partner and letting your partner know about your dietary needs and how they can support you. Choosing calm, stress-free venues that calm your gut and partners who understand your condition can make dating easier. Mutual understanding and support are essential for a successful relationship, so choose flexible and stress-free partners, as they play a massive part in your health and all areas of your life. When dating, it is essential to make thoughtful choices. By prioritising your health and happiness, you can feel empowered and take control of your IBS.

Healthy toilet habits with a footstool

Using a footstool on the toilet can significantly improve your bowel movements. By elevating your feet, you create a more natural angle for your body, reducing strain and discomfort. This position, with your knees above your hips at a 35-degree angle, promotes relaxation and makes it easier for your body to eliminate waste.

Studies using X-rays have shown that squatting straightens out the rectum more effectively. The pressure in the stomach is reduced in this position, indicating less straining. **Try this instead:** if lifestyle changes do not work, set a regular toilet time even when you do not feel the urge. Make it a daily routine for ease. Studies confirm footstools improve posture and reduce straining, particularly with IBS-C, leading to a more comfortable toilet experience. IBS-C or IBS-M individuals should try using a footstool daily to help improve their symptoms and quality of life.

Gentle colon cleansing for IBS relief

For those with IBS-C, which primarily affects the colon, a gentle and natural approach to colon cleansing can provide some relief from abdominal uneasiness. By maintaining a healthy colon, you can ensure regular bowel movements and reduce discomfort associated with IBS. Simple methods like increasing fibre intake, staying hydrated, and incorporating probiotics into your diet can gently cleanse your colon. This approach, focusing on dietary changes and hydration, can improve colon health and relieve IBS symptoms without the need for antibiotics or supplements.

If you have access to a neem tree, you can use its leaves to make a paste that can help cleanse your colon and reduce IBS symptoms. Neem is known for its anti-inflammatory and antibacterial properties, which can help reduce inflammation in the gut and balance gut bacteria. Regular use of neem can promote a healthier digestive system and improve overall gut health.

You can take one ball daily in the morning on an empty stomach. Start with small amounts and see how your body responds. To maintain overall health, it is wise to avoid neem tablets and processed neem powders. Instead, opt for whole foods and natural sources of nutrients whenever possible. This approach gives you all the essential nutrients your body needs in the most natural and easy-to-digest way possible.

Bonus tip: to make neem taste better, mix the paste with honey to reduce the bitterness. You can also combine neem paste with jaggery (unrefined cane sugar) to improve the flavour naturally. Drinking a glass of water right after taking the neem ball helps wash down the strong, bitter taste. Another idea is to blend neem paste into a smoothie with solid flavours like banana or mango to balance the taste. Including a few drops of lemon juice can also help counteract the bitterness.

Neem helps by reducing inflammation in the gut and balancing the gut bacteria, which can reduce symptoms like bloating, gas, and abdominal pain. Regular use can promote a healthier digestive system and improve overall gut health.

Avoid expensive detox teas and try the below two options found in large Asian supermarkets.

Agathi keerai, or hummingbird tree leaves, act as a gentle laxative, helping to clear out your bowels and relieve constipation. The high fibre content aids digestion and keeps your bowel movements regular. The leaves also reduce inflammation in your gut, easing IBS symptoms. They are rich in vitamins and minerals that support good digestion. Including fresh leaves in your diet can help clean your colon, ease IBS symptoms, and keep your digestive system healthy.

Secondly, try consuming Manathakkali, also known as black nightshade spinach. It is helpful for individuals with IBS. Manathakkali calms and heals the stomach lining, reducing pain and discomfort from IBS. It naturally cleanses the colon, helping to remove waste and keep your digestive system clean. The leaves also reduce inflammation in the gut, which eases IBS symptoms. It is rich in vitamins and minerals that support good digestion and helps the body heal. In short, eating Manathakkali can soothe your stomach, clean your colon, and reduce IBS symptoms, making you feel better overall. **Key takeaway:** try including black nightshade spinach, moringa, neem, and hummingbird tree leaves on alternative weeks or each week as natural healers. Eat them as fresh leaves cooked in your meals, and avoid powders or tablets for optimal long-term gut health. These leaves can help regulate digestion, reduce inflammation, cleanse and heal your gut, and provide essential nutrients, which are great for managing IBS.

Reducing chemical exposure at home to help manage IBS

Avoiding chemical household cleaning products entirely is tough, but we can use them less often and for shorter periods. The International Journal of Environmental Sciences & Natural Resources research focuses on "The Dirty Dozen Cleaning Products at Home." These include air fresheners, ammonia, bleach, carpet and upholstery shampoos, dishwasher detergents, drain cleaners, furniture polish, mould and mildew cleaners, oven cleaners, antibacterial cleaners, laundry room products, and toilet bowl cleaners. While essential for cleanliness, these products often contain harmful chemicals.

On average, household cleaning products can contain over 62 toxic chemicals, including harmful substances such as ammonia, coal tar dyes, cocamide DEA, chlorine bleach, DEA (diethanolamine), MEA (monoethanolamine), TEA (triethanolamine), formaldehyde, fragrance (a mix of over 3000 toxic chemicals), glycol ethers, phosphates, triclosan (an antibacterial agent), and sodium borate. Although typically in small amounts in commercial dish detergents, these chemicals can accumulate over time and potentially cause long-term health problems. These chemicals can affect conditions like IBS, potentially causing symptoms like sensitivities.

"Dirty Dozen" refers to everyday household cleaning products that may contain harsh chemicals. For example:

1. Bleach: use vinegar and water instead for cleaning surfaces.
2. Ammonia: use lemon juice and water for a natural cleaner.
3. Air fresheners: opt for essential oils or open windows for fresh air.
4. Disinfectants: choose hydrogen peroxide or alcohol-based cleaners.
5. Antibacterial soaps: use mild, fragrance-free soaps to avoid irritants.
6. Furniture polish: try a mix of olive oil and lemon juice.
7. Carpet cleaners: vacuum regularly and use baking soda to control odours.
8. Laundry detergents: choose fragrance-free, hypoallergenic options.
9. Dishwashing detergents: select natural alternatives without synthetic fragrances.
10. Oven cleaners: use a safer baking soda and vinegar cleaning paste.
11. Mold removers: use vinegar or diluted tea tree oil.
12. All-purpose cleaners: make your own with vinegar, baking soda, and water or orange peel soaked for a week in vinegar and diluted in water.

Choosing natural alternatives and reducing exposure to chemicals can improve overall health. They are also eco-friendly and budget-friendly. Gut health encompasses more than just the food you consume; it is also affected by the products you use in your home.

CHAPTER RECAP:

Healthy microbiome-friendly daily habits can nurture your gut health and overall well-being. Alongside understanding food groups like the 'dirty dozen' and 'clean fifteen', avoiding unnecessary antibiotics to protect your gut bacteria is essential. Seek advice from those with similar experiences, and always cross-check when researching. Prioritise natural remedies over medications whenever possible. Balancing your diet with portion control, incorporating movement, and mindful eating can support gut health. Reading food labels involves checking the position of the IBS trigger foods in the ingredient list and considering the overall nutritional quality for daily consumption.

For travellers and diners, planning ahead and selecting suitable options are key. Lifestyle factors like minimising screen time and practicing gentle colon cleansing can help manage IBS symptoms effectively.

Make changes slowly, focusing on one at a time to see how they affect you. Consistency is critical here, especially with the lifestyle adjustments I have suggested for those with similar conditions. Positivity, nature, and food choices play vital roles in managing symptoms. **Remember**, for IBS-C, stay happy and stay gutsy.

Skip the pricey detox teas and try these natural options from Asian supermarkets. Agathi keerai, known as hummingbird tree leaves, neem leaves, moringa leaves, and manathakkali, known as black nightshade spinach, help cleanse your colon, ease constipation, and reduce gut inflammation. They are full of fibre, vitamins, and minerals supporting digestion. Cook and eat these fresh green leaves regularly for sustained long-term gut health. Adding them to your diet weekly can effectively help manage IBS symptoms as they cleanse and heal your stomach lining.

Give your body time to adapt to any changes. If symptoms persist, it is advisable to seek advice from a healthcare professional, like a dietician, who may recommend a low FODMAP diet. Ensure it is tailored yet diverse nutritionally with portion control to promote a healthy microbiome. Look for natural alternatives to household cleaning products to cut down on toxins that could increase gut sensitivities. If diarrhoea or constipation remains an issue, seek further professional advice. The chapter concentrated on lifestyle practices for promoting a healthy microbiome.

15. Microbiome-Friendly Foods and Recipes

"Everyone thinks of changing the world, but no one thinks of changing himself." — Leo Tolstoy

In Ayurveda and modern science, there is an ongoing study about how dosha imbalances affect the gut. Ayurveda suggests that if doshas are out of balance, they can affect digestion and health, potentially impacting the composition and performance of the gut microbiome bacteria.

However, there is limited scientific proof directly linking dosha imbalances to changes in the gut bacteria. Research looks into how diet, lifestyle, and stress affect dosha balance and impact gut bacteria. Understanding this connection could help better manage health conditions like IBS.

Based on your dosha type identified earlier in the chapter Potential Impact of Body Types on IBS, balancing doshas through lifestyle and diet adjustments is recommended. For example, after taking the dosha quiz we discussed earlier, opt for cooling and nourishing foods like gluten-free whole grains, fruits, and bitter greens if pitta dosha is dominant. **Personal tip:** while websites like Banyan Botanicals focus more on doshas than IBS, personal experimentation has helped me find what works. I have adjusted my diet based on their suggestions, which are explained further.

The dosha dominant diet recommendations below based on dosha type were beneficial for me in handling IBS flare-ups by knowing which food to combine and avoid. This means that if you have IBS-C and experience symptoms similar to mine, your recommended diet might be different. Your body type, or dosha, could be different from mine, and your triggers, including trigger foods, can vary from mine. That is why we are talking about the dosha approach here, as it helps tailor advice to your specific needs, considering factors like your dosha type, to better manage IBS triggers. This tailored approach, lifestyle practices, and meal planning have benefited my IBS-C and lifestyle.

For example, pitta dosha balancing diet recommendations suggested by the Banyan Botanicals dosha quiz were:

"Opt for a diet rich in fresh, whole foods, both cooked and raw, known for their cooling, hearty, and nourishing qualities. This helps to reduce internal heat, alleviate inflammation, balance digestive fire, and ground the body while absorbing excess liquid and oil. Pitta individuals benefit from slowing down and fully engaging with each meal. Consider these additional tips:

Favor Pitta-Pacifying Tastes by choosing foods that are:

Sweet: include grains, fruits, squashes, root vegetables, and fresh dairy products.

Bitter: incorporate bitter greens like kale, dandelion, or collards, along with spices such as cumin and turmeric.

Astringent: choose legumes, vegetables, apples, cranberries, green bananas, and pomegranates."

Personal discovery: although the Banyan Botanicals website focuses more on doshas than IBS, I have discovered what works for me through my experiments. I have decided to remove dairy milk and apples from my diet. However, I still enjoy cheese in moderation for variety and nutrition, with no artificial supplements. I have adjusted my meal plan using the tracker suggestions in the 'Dietary Changes: Meal Planning' section, which suits my IBS-C needs and lifestyle well.

Additional recommendations from Banyan Botanicals based on the Dosa quiz results to *"Reduce Pitta-Aggravating Tastes by moderating foods that are:*

- *Pungent: moderate intake of spicy foods like chilies, radishes, raw garlic, raw onion, and particularly heating spices in oils.*
- *Sour: limit consumption of vinegar, pineapples, grapefruits, and alcohol.*
- *Salty: use salt very sparingly to reduce bloating."*

I adapted the above advice from to fit my IBS-C needs by eliminating alcohol, onion, and garlic (both raw and cooked), including heavy foods such as fried foods from my diet, by replacing them with grilled foods. This calmed the internal digestive fire, preventing inflammation and balancing Agni (digestive fire).

Personal tip: eat fact, NOT fiction. I eat for nutrition, not mere taste. I train my mind and taste buds to crave healthy, tasty food. I make a conscious effort by picturing how uncomfortable and unwell I feel when I consume certain trigger foods, compared to how healthy and happy I could be if I avoid them.

Trying out trendy or extreme diets might leave you needing more essential nutrients. Instead, I take a different approach. I experiment with low FODMAP foods while considering my body's dominant dosha. I monitor how my body reacts, including symptoms, bowel movements, and stool consistency. Based on this, I adjusted my diet by adding a variety of moderately-sized meals. It is a continuous journey as our bodies, circumstances, and age change. Nurture your mind; in return, your body will always do wonders for you.

Superfoods

A superfood is one that is packed with nutrients that are good for your health. They are a vital source of vitamins, minerals, and antioxidants, which can help keep the body strong and healthy. Some examples of superfoods include berries, leafy greens, nuts, and seeds.

When it comes to improving your gut microbiome, the community of bacteria and other microorganisms living in your digestive tract, eating a diet rich in fibre and nutrients is essential. This can support the growth of beneficial bacteria in your gut, enhancing digestion and overall health.

A healthy gut has been associated with enhanced mood and lower obesity rates overall. When your gut functions well, it can help regulate your appetite, metabolism, and mood. Therefore, consuming a diet that promotes a healthy gut can improve your overall well-being and reduce your risk of specific health problems.

Let us look into some traditional superfoods that have been passed down through generations:

1. Amla

It is also known as Indian gooseberry. This small fruit is packed with nutrients like vitamin C, antioxidants, and fibre. It is known for enhancing immunity, supporting digestion, and fostering healthy skin and hair.

A simple recipe could be an amla smoothie:

Blend together chopped Amla with water, some yoghurt, fresh curry leaves, a touch of honey, and a handful of spinach for a nourishing and refreshing beverage. Avoid ice and drink at room temperature to enhance nutrient absorption and facilitate smoother bowel movements.

Fermented Amla recipe option 2:

Would you like to try something new? Refer to the image below:

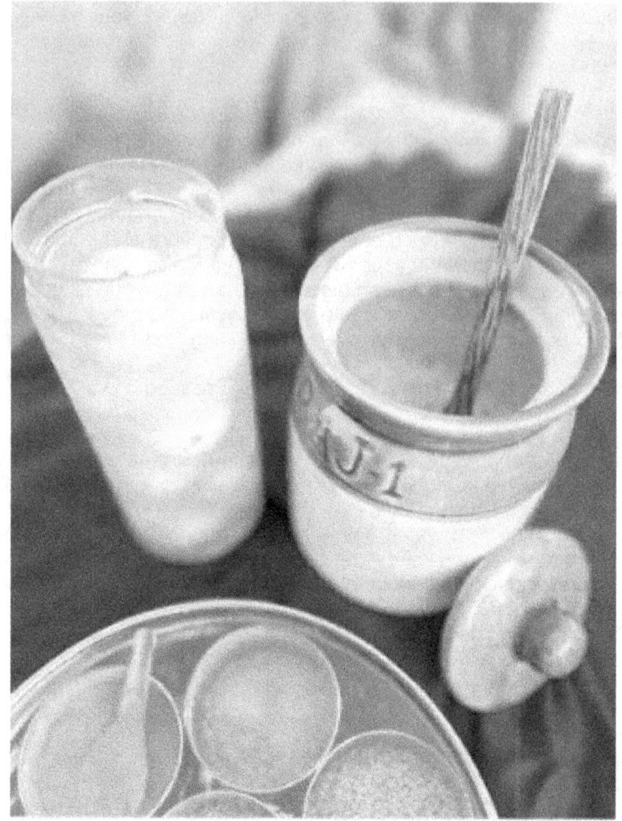

Preparation, arrangement and photography of fermented amla by Jan Nallathamby

Put a few amla fruits in a clean glass bottle. Add some fresh filtered water, a pinch of rock salt, a bit of turmeric, and a tiny bit of fenugreek. Shake it well and close the lid tightly. Let it sit at room temperature for about a week or longer if it is cold. If you are sensitive to spicy food, such as a pittta dominant dosha, skip adding slit green chillies when fermenting and skip garlic if it is an IBS trigger. Taste it using a dry spoon to know if it is ready, and keep it in the fridge to stop it from fermenting further. It can stay suitable for up to 6 months if you seal the lid tightly. Have one big amla or two smaller ones every day. It makes for a tasty snack or side dish. These small, consistent, healthy efforts save expensive long-term medical bills in fixing microbiome health.

2. Moringa

It is a nutrient-dense plant native to parts of Africa and Asia. It is rich in vitamins, minerals, and antioxidants, making it a great addition to any diet. Moringa has been linked to improved energy levels, better digestion, and reduced inflammation. Try stirring moringa in oil, ginger, dried red chillies, and salt until it is wilted. Add desiccated fresh coconut and serve. Replace coconut with cooked chicken, shrimp, tofu, or eggs to make it a more substantial dish. For a nutty flavour, sprinkle toasted sesame seeds or chopped nuts on top before serving to enhance texture and taste.

Tip: skip the powdered and tablet moringa; opt for fresh moringa in Asian supermarkets worldwide. Eat fresh moringa leaves to boost your gut health for the optimal results. Rinse fresh moringa leaves under running water after soaking them briefly with a pinch of rock sea salt and turmeric powder. This ensures thorough cleansing, allowing water to penetrate the leaves and remove potential pesticides.

3. Bitter gourd

Also known as bitter melon, it is a vegetable with a distinct bitter taste. Despite its taste, bitter gourd is incredibly nutritious, containing vitamins, minerals, and antioxidants. It is recognised for regulating blood sugar levels, improving digestion, and boosting immunity. For a healthy recipe, try stuffed bitter gourd by scooping out the seeds, stuff the bitter gourd with a mixture of spiced lentils or ground meat, and steam or bake until tender.

Alternatively, marinate washed bitter gourd slices in sea salt and tamarind puree water for 10 minutes, then rinse them before cooking to remove bitterness. Adding ginger and mild spices topped with fresh coconut milk can balance bitterness and choosing younger gourds. This can reduce some solid bitter taste, as bitter gourd flavours differ depending on the type.

4. Ragi millet

It is also known as finger millet, a type of millet grain that has been a staple in South Indian cuisine for centuries. It is wholly gluten-free for your gut and also comes in powder form. As a complex carbohydrate, ragi is digested more slowly than simple carbohydrates, providing a sustained release of energy, thereby reducing appetite for healthy weight management and energy release. It is full of fibre, calcium, iron, minerals, and antioxidants, all of which help keep your gut healthy, aid weight management, regulate blood sugar levels, and improve bone health. The fibre in ragi helps you have regular bowel movements and encourages the growth of good bacteria in your gut. Ragi also has prebiotics, which feeds the good bacteria in your gut and keeps them strong. Eating ragi regularly as part of a balanced diet can help you digest food better and keep your gut healthy.

Consider making ragi porridge or ragi malt for a nutritious and versatile recipe. Start by dissolving ragi flour in filtered tap water to form a thick, smooth paste. Add this to a pot of boiling water, stirring until thickened, and then add some powdered jaggery for a sweet taste. When it starts bubbling, it is ready. Allow it to cool down, then blend the ragi malt drink until it is smooth and frothy. The image below shows the top with overnight soaked and peeled nuts such as almonds. This dish is not only filling but also rich in iron, which is essential during periods for women, helping balance hormones differently for women with IBS and easing symptoms. It is part of a balanced diet rich in calcium and fibre to help maintain regular bowel movements. For a savoury twist, swap jaggery powder with yoghurt once it cools, making it a refreshing summer drink or garnished with fruits for extra taste and nutrients. The versatility of ragi millet in recipes can inspire you to get creative in the kitchen and rejoice in the nutritional health benefits of this traditional superfood, bringing a sense of joy and satisfaction to your cooking experience.

These traditional superfoods, including ragi millet, are not only nutrient-dense and provide various health benefits, but they are also affordable. This affordability makes them excellent additions to a balanced diet that supports a healthy microbiome, especially for individuals with IBS. Millets, mainly, are rich in soluble fibre, which is crucial for reducing gastrointestinal issues. Millets, often called a 'poor man's crop ', are grown in marginal environments and thrive with minimal water. They have been re-branded as nutri-cereals and intelligent foods, valued for their contributions to gut health. Ragi millet, in particular, plays a significant role in supporting farmers and promoting health-oriented businesses. By incorporating these affordable and nutrient-dense superfoods into your diet, you can feel empowered and included in the movement towards better health and a healthier planet. Improve meal diversity with a blend of various millets to maximise the nutritional benefits of each variety.

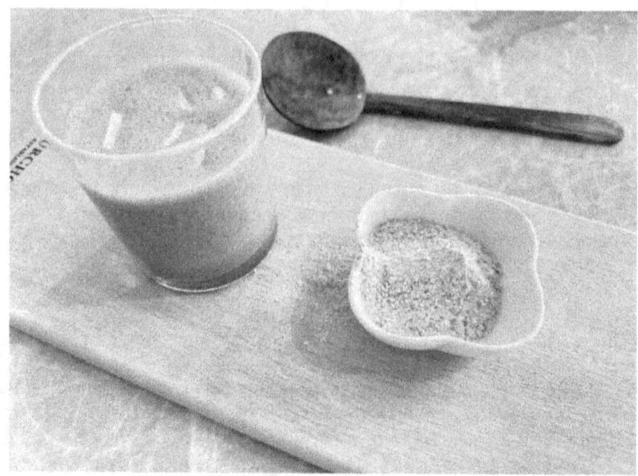

Preparation, arrangement and photography of ragi malt by Jan Nallathamby

Ragi millet can help manage IBS symptoms like constipation and diarrhoea because it is fibre-rich and might have prebiotic effects. For those with constipation, ragi's fibre can help keep bowels moving smoothly. For those with diarrhoea, ragi's soluble fibre might help soak up excess water and make stools firmer. It could also help balance out for those with mixed symptoms. But pay attention to how your body reacts to ragi, and if it does not sit well with you, avoid it or have it in small amounts.

For more easy and quick millet recipes, visit the YouTube channel "Skinny Recipes" and select the ones that align with your personal tastes to support your gut health requirements.

CHAPTER RECAP:

Ayurveda and modern science are studying how dosha imbalances affect gut health. Ayurveda suggests that imbalanced doshas can impact digestion and gut bacteria, but scientific proof is still limited. Researchers are exploring how diet, lifestyle, and stress, which influence doshas, also affect gut bacteria. Understanding this connection could help manage IBS better.

Your dosha type, identified in the "Potential Impact of Body Types on IBS" chapter, guides diet and lifestyle adjustments. For example, if you have a dominant pitta dosha, choose cooling foods like gluten-free grains, fruits, and bitter greens that will help you feel better and aid the growth of good gut bacteria over the long term. Experimentation based on Banyan Botanicals' suggestions or other similar sources can help tailor your diet to manage IBS symptoms.

Avoid overly spicy, sour, and salty foods. Replace dairy milk with alternatives and avoid foods that cause discomfort. Track symptoms to adjust your diet continually. Include superfoods like amla, moringa, bitter gourd, and ragi millet, including other similar millets, to support gut health and manage IBS. Be open to exploring natural foods over various medicines that might cause other side effects in the long term.

To nourish your microbiome, prioritise hydrating foods like cucumber and include fibre-rich options by including fruits, vegetables, whole grains, and legumes in your daily diet, but in moderation. It suggests combining pulses with cumin and carom (ajwain) seed water for improved digestion and reduced gas. Pay attention to the 'Dirty Dozen' and 'Clean Fifteen' lists when making food choices, as discussed in the earlier chapter. These foods foster the growth of beneficial bacteria in the gut. Avoid processed foods, excessive sugar, and artificial additives, as they can harm your microbiome and disrupt gut balance.

Complex carbohydrates like millets, quinoa, and brown rice are better than simple carbohydrates because they digest slowly, giving you steady energy and helping your gut health. These foods contain fibre that nourishes beneficial bacteria in your gut, supporting a diverse and healthy gut microbiota and promoting regular bowel movements.

In addition, incorporate fermented foods in moderation, like yoghurt, kombucha, kefir, sauerkraut, and kimchi, which are rich in probiotics that boost healthy gut bacteria. Try prebiotic foods that contain fibres that feed the beneficial bacteria in your gut, like oats and bananas, to nourish the good gut bacteria. Consider avoiding or substituting high FODMAP foods like onions, garlic, and prebiotics if they trigger your IBS symptoms. Refer to the 'Meal Planning for IBS: Tips and Tricks' chapter for alternatives.

Focusing on a balanced diet and understanding your body's specific needs can help you better manage IBS and improve overall gut health.

It is encouraged to consume natural foods and eat facts, not fiction.

Practical Guidance and Strategies

"My destination is no longer a place, rather a new way of seeing." — Marcel Proust

This chapter is a beacon of empowerment, offering practical guidance and strategies to support those with IBS on their journey towards better digestive health. Whether you are looking to make dietary changes through meal planning tips specifically designed for individuals with IBS to help reduce symptoms, establish morning and night routines for gut health, or manage stress and incorporate exercise for IBS relief, the suggestions discussed in this chapter can be tailored to address the needs of individuals with IBS.

From tips and tricks for meal planning tailored to IBS to stress management techniques and the profound impact of exercise on gut health, each section provides actionable insights to help those with IBS.

Here are the main types of treatments for IBS in simple terms:

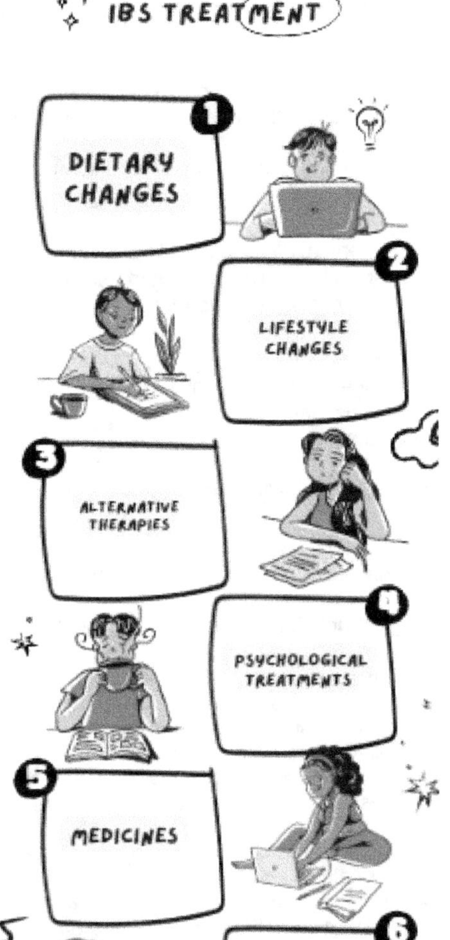

Self-created image by Jan Nallathamby 'IBS treatment types' content from NIDDK

1. Dietary changes:
- A low FODMAP diet is achieved by avoiding foods that cause gas and bloating.
- High-fibre diet by eating more fibre to help with bowel movements.
- Avoid triggering foods by avoiding foods that worsen symptoms, like caffeine, alcohol, and fatty foods.

2. Lifestyle changes:
- Exercise where regular physical activity helps with bowel function and stress.

- Stress management activities like yoga, meditation, and deep breathing can reduce stress.

3. Alternative therapies:
- Acupuncture is where some individuals find relief through this traditional practice.
- Probiotics that help balance gut bacteria. Use artificial supplements if natural foods prove insufficient.
- Herbal remedies, such as peppermint oil, can reduce symptoms.

4. Psychological treatments:
- Cognitive behavioural therapy (CBT) helps manage stress and anxiety related to IBS.
- Hypnotherapy uses hypnosis to reduce gut-related anxiety and improve gut function.
- Mindfulness and relaxation techniques help reduce stress levels.

5. Medicines:
- Antispasmodics help with gut muscle cramps.
- Laxatives for those with constipation.
- Antidiarrheals for those with diarrhoea.
- Antidepressants of low doses can help with pain and gut issues.
- IBS-C and chronic constipation medicines like lubiprostone and linaclotide.

6. Education and support:
- Support groups by talking to others with IBS can provide emotional support and practical advice.
- Education and learning about IBS help in managing the condition better

Combining the treatments mentioned above often yields favourable results. Starting with options 1, 2, and 6 above is a practical way to address the issue. Suppose those methods do not bring the desired results. In that case, it is crucial to collaborate with a healthcare provider, such as a gastroenterologist or a registered dietitian, to explore other options. Opt for natural food remedies over options like option 5 whenever possible to prioritise long-term gut microbiome health. Given the complexity of IBS, starting with simple dietary and lifestyle changes is ideal to minimise potential side effects in the long run.

Subsequent chapters explore various dietary components, including protein sources, dairy alternatives, and carbohydrates. They emphasise the importance of balanced nutrition and understanding food labels, encouraging a focus on healthier options.

Moreover, the content highlights maintaining a healthy weight through mindful eating and understanding body mass index (BMI), which will be discussed further under the chapter 'Exercise and it's Impact on Gut Health'. It also advises tracking symptoms and dietary changes to monitor their long-term effects, encouraging the reader to take an active role in their health management.

The text provides tailored dietary recommendations for specific digestive issues. For constipation, it suggests gradually increasing fibre intake and incorporating powdered flaxseeds daily to aid bowel movement. For diarrhoea, staying hydrated, reducing caffeine and alcohol consumption, and avoiding trigger foods are recommended.

The chapter also touches upon the potential benefits of probiotics for digestive health, suggesting a cautious approach when trying probiotic supplements and monitoring their effects over time.

It offers comprehensive dietary guidance tailored to individual digestive issues, emphasising the importance of listening to one's body and making informed nutritional choices. This empowers the reader to take control of their health and ensures they understand the impact of their dietary decisions.

16. Dietary Changes: Meal Planning

"Experience is the name so many people give to their mistakes." — Francis Scott Fitzgerald

To manage IBS symptoms effectively, focus on dietary adjustments like increasing fibre intake through fruits, vegetables, whole grains, and legumes. Hydration is vital; drinking plenty of water softens stool and supports regular bowel movements. Identify trigger foods like fatty or spicy items, caffeine, and alcohol, then avoid them to minimise symptoms. Choose smaller, more frequent meals to avoid overloading your digestive system. Consulting healthcare providers or dietitians for personalised dietary plans tailored to individual symptoms and triggers can enhance effective management. These plans should incorporate various ingredients across cuisines to add diversity and promote gut microbiome growth. This approach ensures holistic support for managing IBS symptoms and optimising overall digestive health.

Incorporate food and symptoms tracking into meal planning

Keeping a food and symptom diary while making dietary changes can help track what has been beneficial. Making one change at a time is ideal to better understand what works. These tools, suitable for new and long-term IBS managers, enable individuals to identify food triggers and plan meals accordingly, improving their ability to manage their health journey effectively.

Seeking guidance from a dietitian promptly can significantly benefit those managing IBS. The low FODMAP diet, which involves reducing fermentable carbohydrates like onion and wheat to ease digestive discomfort, outlined in these trackers alongside meal diversity and portion control, has aided in my IBS-C management as a lived expert. I have found that continuous learning and adaptation are essential, especially while awaiting further advancements in microbiome research. It is vital to refine our approach based on individual experiences. This professional guidance can provide reassurance and support in your IBS management journey.

Personal tip: find balance and avoid making strict plans. Add more joy to your day and expect occasional slip-ups. Instead of dwelling on mistakes, view them as opportunities to learn and move forward positively, fostering a sense of encouragement and optimism.

The below resources provide valuable tools for managing IBS and understanding the FODMAP diet, which helps reduce symptoms. The IBS tracker, food diary, and symptom tracker help individuals monitor their diet and symptoms to identify triggers. The FODMAP diet food guide and low/high FODMAP grocery list offer practical guidance on foods to include and avoid. With the IBS diet food list and grocery list, individuals can easily plan meals that support gut health. The complete FODMAP shopping list provides a comprehensive overview of low and high FODMAP foods, facilitating grocery shopping for those following the diet. Lastly, the FODMAP IBS food list and low FODMAP treats guide individuals in creating nutritious meal plans that promote gut health while enjoying delicious treats that are gentle on the stomach. These resources empower individuals to take control of their diet and manage their IBS effectively, instilling a sense of empowerment and control.

- IBS Tracker, Food Diary, Allergy, Medicine and Supplement Tracking Sheet, Diet Tracker, Meal Planner, Daily Health Planner, Symptom Tracker by Etsy seller FRGLMAMA <u>click here</u> or refer to the chapter 'Additional Resources' for the full link.

- FODMAP Diet Food Guide, Low and High FODMAP Grocery List, IBS Food List, Food Chart, Nutrition Dietitian Worksheet (Digital Printable) by Etsy seller LearningHealthCo <u>click here</u> or refer to the chapter 'Additional Resources' for the full link.

- IBS Diet, Irritable Bowel Syndrome, Food List, Grocery List, Food Guide, What To Eat, What Not To Eat, Gut Health Nutrition, PDF Download by Etsy seller TheSecretPrintables <u>click here</u> or refer to the chapter 'Additional Resources' for the full link.

- Complete FODMAP shopping list - Low FODMAP and high FODMAP food list - FODMAP diet grocery list – FODMAP chart for irritable bowel syndrome by Etsy seller NutriWellness click here or refer to the chapter 'Additional Resources' for the full link.

- FODMAP IBS Food List and Low FODMAP Treats, Food Chart Nutrition Guide for IBS Meal Plan and Gut Health, Gluten-Free Diet Meal Prep Grocery by Etsy seller TheMichellicious click here or refer to the chapter 'Additional Resources' for the full link.

The next step is to explore these resources further and determine which ones align well with your IBS needs and preferences. Consider reviewing each resource in more detail to understand how it can support you in managing your IBS and following a FODMAP diet with various cuisines in moderation, eliminating only the high-trigger foods and enjoying the rest. Consider consulting with a healthcare provider or registered dietitian for personalised guidance and recommendations tailored to your needs.

CHAPTER RECAP:

In managing IBS, focus on dietary adjustments like increasing fibre intake and staying hydrated. Identify trigger foods and avoid them while opting for smaller, frequent meals. Utilise food and symptom tracking tools to monitor your diet and IBS symptoms, making one change at a time for better understanding. Seek guidance from a dietitian promptly where results seem delayed, and embrace the low FODMAP diet with a blend of meal diversity and mindful portion control. To improve your digestive health, consider eliminating high-IBS-trigger foods like alcohol, onions, garlic, apples, and pears. These triggers can differ for each person. Therefore, tailor your diet to meet your needs for improved digestive health.

Explore the provided resources to find tools that align with your IBS needs and preferences. If necessary, consult with healthcare professionals for personalised guidance. Continuous learning and adaptation are vital in refining your approach, so never give up. Keep trying and believing.

17. Morning and Night Routine for Gut Health and Well-being

"Don't educate your children to be rich. Educate them to be happy, so they know the value of things, not the price." — Victor Hugo

Easy-to-follow morning routine habits for gut health

Morning routine habit 1: set the intention for the day

For example, an intention for the day could be, 'Today, I choose to nourish my body with foods that support my gut health and bring me comfort.' By setting this intention, you are affirming your commitment to self-care and making choices that prioritise your well-being and the health of your microbiome.

Consider switching from coffee and understand your reasons, whether to ease IBS symptoms or improve sleep. Knowing your motivation can help you stay committed. Instead, start your day with warm water mixed with two teaspoons of organic, unpasteurised apple cider vinegar (ACV) on an empty stomach, or opt for herbal teas. Avoid dairy if it triggers your IBS symptoms, and aim for warm beverages to support bowel movements. ACV's probiotics can help restore gut balance, promote digestion, and reduce bloating. However, consult a healthcare provider if you have pre-existing conditions before using ACV on an empty stomach.

Gradually reduce your coffee intake or switch to smaller cups. Consume ACV in moderation, diluted with warm water, three times a week to prevent throat and stomach irritation. ACV has improved my bowel regularity, but results can vary for each person. **Personal tip:** I drink a glass of warm water on an empty stomach first thing in the morning to help with bowel regularity. Also, spend 5-10 minutes in the morning sunlight to get natural vitamin D, essential for bone health, the immune system, and overall well-being. Morning sunlight also boosts serotonin production, which helps you feel happy and positive. These habits can support overall digestive health, especially for those with IBS.

If you are feeling adventurous, start with 100 ml and up to 200 ml per day of homemade white ash gourd juice, also called winter melon or wax gourd juice. It is usually less likely to trigger IBS symptoms when drunk on an empty stomach. It is a hydrating and soothing drink, often used for its cooling properties in summer. However, everyone is different, so pay attention to how your body reacts.

Ending your shower with 1-2 minutes of cold water can help manage IBS bloating. The cold water can reduce inflammation and improve circulation, which might help with bloating. It also gives your body a nice wake-up, boosting your mood and energy levels. This can make you feel better when coping with IBS symptoms and support your digestive health.

Morning routine habit 2: oil pulling

After morning habit 1, try oil pulling, which was previously discussed in the chapter' Lifestyle Practices to Promote a Healthy Microbiome'.

Morning routine habit 3: write a 5- minute daily journal with a stress log

While doing habit 2 above, establish a routine by dedicating a specific daily time for mindfulness and journaling. Being consistent with these exercises is critical to seeing long-term benefits. When you journal, be honest to accurately identify patterns and triggers. It can also be helpful to share your mindfulness and journaling experiences with a support group or therapist for additional guidance.

Daily, write down how you feel, any stress you are experiencing, and how it might affect your gut. Reflect on moments of gratitude and positive experiences to cultivate a positive mindset. When you encounter stressful situations, jot down how you handled them and any physical symptoms you experienced. Reflect on what coping strategies worked well and what did not.

Tips: were the below potential triggers for your IBS symptoms:

- Recent life events?
- Changes in routine during holidays?
- Specific foods in your diet?
- Note if symptoms happen at specific times of the day?

Remember not to judge yourself for your thoughts, feelings, or symptoms. Start with short journaling sessions and gradually increase the time if you feel comfortable to avoid overwhelming yourself. Address emotional triggers constructively in your journaling to better manage your IBS symptoms.

Incorporating mindfulness exercises and journaling into your daily routine can strengthen the connection between your gut and brain, helping you manage stress and better understand your IBS triggers. This approach can lead to improved symptom management and overall well-being.

You can make journaling more fun using tools like the Tummy Trouble Tracker and cute happy gut stickers. These creative tools make tracking your symptoms feel less like a chore and more personal. Set aside time each week to look over your tracked data. Look for any patterns or connections between your symptoms, what triggers them, and your daily habits. Try adding it to your morning routine as a regular habit to make tracking easier. For those with long-term IBS, using colourful stickers or emojis to show symptom severity each day can make tracking more interesting. Assign different colours or emojis to show how bad your symptoms are so you can quickly see how they change over time.

- Tummy Trouble Tracker by Etsy seller StardustStickers click here or refer to the chapter 'Additional Resources' for the full link.
- 35 Cute Happy Gut/IBS Planner Stickers by Etsy seller HappyCutieStudio click here or refer to the chapter 'Additional Resources' for the full link.

If you face challenges after trying these self-management approaches, consider discussing the tracked data with a healthcare provider to explore further treatment options tailored to your needs. Use this information to make informed decisions about dietary adjustments, stress management techniques, or lifestyle modifications, as each day or week can be different, calling for frequent review and adjustment to diet and lifestyle over the days, weeks, and months.

Simple dietary adjustments often reduce IBS symptoms, while prioritising relaxation and stress reduction remains paramount. Incorporating mindfulness exercises and journaling into your daily routine can strengthen the gut-brain connection, manage stress, and better understand your IBS triggers. This approach can lead to improved symptom management and overall well-being.

If you are still having trouble after trying the self-management approach, consider discussing the tracked data with a healthcare provider to gain insights and explore further treatment options that fit your needs.

Morning routine habit 4: quick 5-minute diaphragmatic breathing and 2 minutes body scan meditation

To incorporate a calming morning habit, try a quick 5-minute diaphragmatic breathing exercise to soothe your limbic system. Sit comfortably and close your eyes. Take slow, deep breaths, inhaling gently through your nose for a count of four, holding for four, and then exhaling through your mouth for four. Repeat this cycle to reduce stress and promote relaxation. Starting your day calmly and positively can help support your IBS management.

Lie down or sit comfortably and close your eyes. Slowly direct your focus to each part of your body, beginning from your toes and progressing upward to your head. Recognise any tension or discomfort and breathe deeply into those areas to promote relaxation. Spend 2 minutes on this exercise to boost your body awareness and encourage relaxation.

Morning routine habit 5: stretching exercises for 7 minutes followed by 2 minutes weights and 5 minutes yoga

Try easy stretches like touching your toes, reaching up high, and bending to the side to loosen tension in your abdominal area. You can also do the Japanese Radio Taiso exercise routine for about 7.46 minutes. Click here. It is on YouTube under ラジオ体操 第一 第二 首 by album-chat, published on 20 August 2016 by albums-chat, which includes a series of light stretches and movements designed to get your blood flowing and make you more flexible. This is a game changer since it is quick and suitable for all fitness levels.

After that, do a 2-minute arm weight lift to strengthen your muscles and get your blood flowing, and follow it with a 5-minute yoga session. In this yoga, click here It is on YouTube under 'Yoga for women! #yogateacher #yogawithkamya #onlineyogaclass #shortsvideo #yogaforweightloss #fyp' published 1 December 2023 by yogawithkamya_, the Malasana walk massages your stomach and help bowel movements, while butterfly flaps loosen your tummy muscles and can support better bowel movements which is particularly ideal for IBS-C symptoms.

Yoga also relaxes you, reduces stress, and improves digestion with gentle moves and breathing exercises. Doing this routine in the morning can ease IBS-C symptoms by improving gut movement and relaxing your abdominal region. It wakes your body, aids digestion, and reduces bloating and discomfort from IBS.

These exercises activate digestion, lower bloating and abdominal tension associated with IBS and improve overall gut health. Stretching eases tummy tension, while weightlifting strengthens your core for better bowel movements. Making this routine part of your day prepares your body for whatever comes and can lessen IBS troubles.

Starting your day like this helps manage IBS better. It makes it easier to stick to a healthy morning routine that reduces IBS flare-ups and contributes to overall well-being. Stretching, strength training and yoga only take 14 minutes, which is perfect for those short on time. Doing different physical variations in short bursts yet consistently in the morning helps improve gut health and build resistance over time.

Making this routine part of your daily balanced exercise regime helps your body prepare for the day ahead and keeps your digestive system active. By starting your day with these exercises, you build a healthy, proactive way to manage IBS. It is easier to stick to a consistent morning routine that is good for your digestive health.

Morning routine habit 6: matcha or chia in coconut water with fermented amla and probiotic supplement

Starting your day with a refreshing blend of plain matcha tea or chia seeds soaked in coconut water with fermented amla is a fantastic way to kickstart your morning and support your health soon after habit 5 above. Matcha, a green tea powder, is packed with antioxidants and can give you a gentle boost in energy without the typical jitters that come with coffee. Chia seeds are abundant in dietary fibre and omega-3 fatty acids, essential for a healthy digestive system and can help regulate bowel movements. Coconut water is hydrating and contains electrolytes, making it an excellent option for rehydrating after a night's sleep.

Adding fermented amla (one to two fruits of amla), as discussed in the chapter Microbiome-Friendly Foods and Recipes, to this mix provides additional benefits for your gut health. Amla, also known as Indian gooseberry, is a plentiful source of vitamin C and other nutrients that aid digestion and support immune function. When fermented, amla becomes even more potent, as fermentation enhances its probiotic properties, promoting a healthy balance of gut bacteria.

This morning drink hydrates you and provides a nutritional boost that can help support your digestive system. The combination of matcha or chia seeds in coconut water and fermented amla delivers a blend of antioxidants, fibre, and probiotics that can aid digestion, reduce bloating, and reduce symptoms of IBS. The gentle energy from a cup of warm matcha can assist in maintaining alertness and focus throughout the day without experiencing the crash often associated with sugary or caffeinated cold drinks.

Incorporating this morning habit into your routine nourishes your body. It takes proactive steps to support your digestive health, including managing IBS symptoms and improving overall well-being.

Consider taking a probiotic gut health tablet daily with breakfast. I started with the lowest dosage of 20 billion CFU live-friendly bacteria and took it for nine months straight. **Remember** to take breaks every three months before continuing. This can assist in preserving a healthy equilibrium of gut bacteria, but always listen to your body and see how you feel. Also, it is a good idea to consult your pharmacist or doctor if you plan to continue the probiotic supplement for an extended period. Since these are probiotic tablets, there are typically no proven side effects if taken continuously. I have noticed feeling less groggy, especially with IBS-C symptoms, since adding the probiotic supplement to my daily morning routine.

Easy-to-follow night routine habits for gut health

Night routine habit 1: green tea
Enjoy a cup of green tea in the evening or night. Green tea is abundant in antioxidants and can support digestion. It also has a calming effect, helping you wind down before bed.

Night routine habit 2: belly oiling

Before going to bed, try massaging your belly button with half a teaspoon of room-temperature castor oil in circular motions daily. Start with a few days gap and continue daily if it suits you. This can help relax your abdominal muscles, improve digestion, and support better bowel movements. **Remember** to clean and dry the naval area the following day.

Night routine habit 3: nutrient and hydration check
Ensure you have had a balanced intake of nuts, greens, yoghurt, flax seeds, overnight-soaked almonds, and fermented foods throughout the day. These foods are great for your gut health. Make sure you have consumed an adequate amount of warm water throughout the day. Staying hydrated is important for digestion. A handy flask gets the intake of warm water sorted throughout the day, aiding in regular bowel movements.

Night routine habit 4: light early dinner
Eat a light dinner early in the evening before sunset. This allows your digestive system enough time to digest food before bedtime. Refrain from heavy, fatty, or spicy foods that might cause discomfort, and eliminate alcohol to help manage IBS symptoms more quickly.

Night routine habit 5: loose nightwear
Wearing loose clothes at night helps manage IBS bloating. Tight garments can press on your stomach and make bloating worse. Loose clothes allow your stomach to relax and give it room to breathe, making you more comfortable and reducing bloating. Also, being comfortable at night can help you sleep better, which is excellent for your gut health.

Night routine habit 6: reflect on daily routine
At the end of the day, take a moment to reflect on your morning and night routine habits discussed in this chapter. Think about what you ate, how much water you drank, and how you feel. This can help you stay mindful of your gut health and make necessary adjustments with IBS trigger foods and lifestyle changes.

Adding these morning and night habits to your night routine actively supports your digestive system and promotes overall well-being. Consistency is vital, and making these practices a regular part of your night will help you enjoy optimal results over time.

CHAPTER RECAP:

Consistency in morning and night routines is crucial for gut health and overall well-being. Begin your day with a positive intention, such as nourishing your body with gut-friendly foods. Drink warm water with organic apple cider vinegar to stimulate digestion and improve bowel movement. Spend 5 minutes journaling about your feelings, stress, and IBS triggers, using creative tools like the Tummy Trouble Tracker and happy gut stickers to make tracking more engaging.

Incorporate a short exercise routine with 7 minutes of stretching, 2 minutes of weight lifting, and 5 minutes of yoga to improve digestion and reduce bloating. Start your day with a healthy drink of matcha or chia seeds in coconut water with fermented amla to boost antioxidants, fibre, and probiotics. Consider taking a probiotic supplement with breakfast.

Enjoy a cup of green tea to aid digestion and promote relaxation in the evening. Massage your belly button with castor oil before bed to relax your abdominal muscles and support better bowel movements. Ensure you have had a balanced intake of nutrients and stay hydrated throughout the day. Eat a light dinner early to aid digestion and reduce IBS symptoms. Finally, reflect on your day, noting your food intake and how you feel, to stay mindful of your gut health and make necessary adjustments. Consistency in these simple yet effective habits will support you in managing IBS and promoting a healthy gut, leading to overall well-being for those with IBS.

18. Meal Planning for IBS: Tips and Tricks

"The less one has to do, the less time one finds to do it in." — Lord Chesterfield

Meal planning involves mindful eating based on science and nutrition, not just taste and emotions. It is about making smart food choices, whether eating out or packing meals for the day.

Utilise tracking data to adjust your meal plans and identify patterns in your IBS symptoms. Practical tips can make meal planning more manageable, like preparing meals in advance and choosing convenient, healthy options while avoiding trigger foods.

IBS meal planning tips and tricks

This chapter offers versatile solutions for managing IBS for all types.

For salads, mix up a handful of iceberg, spinach, and rocket for a fibre-rich meal while adding moringa leaves to your diet often. **Bonus tip:** including vegetables and salads in every meal is essential for balanced nutrition and promoting regular bowel movements, especially for individuals with IBS-C. This approach has personally helped me manage my symptoms effectively. Adding fresh mint, coriander, freshly sprouted microgreens or celery to soups and smoothies can help soothe the stomach and enhance the taste.

Consider incorporating homemade immunity gut shots into your routine. Keep your spice usage minimal to avoid triggering symptoms, and experiment with cucumber, coconut, and legumes with asafoetida for better digestion and less gas.

When it comes to snacks, opt for fibre-rich options like fresh dates, figs, and pistachios in moderation, as figs contain fructose that might be malabsorbed. Avoid high-sugar snacks and instead go for low-FODMAP candies, dark chocolate or fresh fruits.

Choose lactose-free or plant-based milk options and sweeteners like stevia or monk fruit for beverages. Experiment with different honey options, focusing on low FODMAP content and rawness.

Limit fresh fruit intake to three portions daily, focusing on whole fruits rather than juices or smoothies for better fibre intake.

Substitute fast food with fresh, minimally processed options, and be mindful of salt and sugar content. Experiment with garlic and onion substitutes to add flavour without triggering symptoms.

Remember to keep hydrated with warm water and regularly move after meals to support healthy digestion. These simple steps are often overlooked but can make a big difference in gut health. Make sure to take time to relax and unwind, as stress can worsen the symptoms of IBS.

Incorporating fermented foods daily, like amla pickles, kimchi, and kombucha, into your diet can support gut health. Consistency is key, so include small portions of fermented foods daily.

Mixing the gluten-free sauce with water to reduce it's salt content can help manage IBS bloating. Too much salt can cause your body to hold onto water, leading to bloating. By diluting your sauce, you lower the salt intake, which can help keep your stomach from feeling too full and uncomfortable. This simple trick helps make meals easier on your digestive system.

Choosing foods listed in the WHO's 'Dirty Dozen,' such as berries, spinach, and tomatoes, and those from the 'clean fifteen' we discussed can help manage IBS by reducing pesticide exposure that can worsen gut sensitivity. Alternatively, washing these foods thoroughly, unless certified organic, before cooking with a solution like vinegar and water can also help remove pesticide residues to some extent, ensuring a cleaner and safer option for gut health. This mindful approach to food selection supports digestive wellness and promotes overall well-being by reducing exposure to harmful chemicals.

Microgreens

Sprouting micro green seeds at home is a fantastic way to boost your fibre intake, vital for managing IBS. Seeds like alfalfa, broccoli, red amaranth, mung bean, lentil, and chia are packed with fibre, aiding in regulating bowel movements and supporting gut health. These sprouts are gentler on digestion and pack more vitamin C, B vitamins, and iron compared to unsprouted seeds.

By soaking the seeds overnight and then rinsing them twice daily in a dark, cloth-covered spot, fresh sprouts will be ready to enhance your meals in just a few days. **Personal tip:** the microgreen sprouts seed pack in the snack bowl pictured below, alongside steamed yellow bell peppers and lentils, are available on Amazon. Click here under 'Verdant Republic Microgreens Salad Seeds Mix | Fawn Collection- 5 Seeds Mix Packs | High Germination & Easy to Sprout | Over 16 Vegetable & Herbs Varieties incl Broccoli, Radish, Kale'. Check the 'Additional Resources' chapter for the complete link. This mix includes five seed packs with a high germination rate and is easy to sprout. It features over 16 vegetable and herb varieties, including broccoli, radish, and kale. It can be found under the product name mentioned above.

Adding micro-green sprouts to your meals is a simple way to boost your fibre intake, aiding digestion and potentially easing IBS symptoms. These sprouts are versatile and can be incorporated into salads, sandwiches, and dishes. **Remember** to maintain hydration by drinking ample water alongside fibre-rich foods for optimal digestive health.

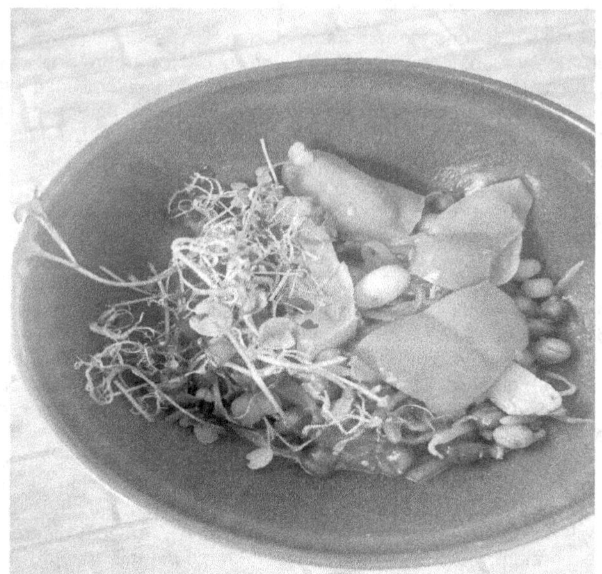

Preparation, arrangement and photography of home sprouted micro green snack bowl by Jan Nallathamby

Gut immunity shots

Immunity gut shots, when homemade, can help manage IBS by boosting your digestive health and immune system with nutrients like vitamin C, zinc, and probiotics. These shots are small but packed with probiotics and nutrients that support a healthy gut flora. For instance, you can easily create a turmeric ginger gut shot by blending fresh turmeric, ginger, lemon juice, and a pinch of black pepper. Turmeric and ginger have anti-inflammatory properties that could reduce symptoms of IBS, such as bloating and discomfort. Regularly taking these shots can improve digestion and strengthen your immunity, making your gut more resilient and healthy. Moderation is critical, as too much can aggravate stomach irritation.

To further enhance immunity for IBS, include incorporating probiotic-rich foods like yoghurt and kefir into your diet, regular exercise to stimulate the immune system, and prioritising quality sleep to allow the body to rest and repair. Immune-boosting foods like citrus fruits and leafy greens can supply vital vitamins and minerals that promote gut health.

Quick and mild meals

Keeping your meals simple by using no more than five ingredients and limiting spices to four or fewer can be beneficial for managing IBS. This approach reduces the risk of triggering IBS symptoms, as complex dishes with many ingredients and herbs can be tricky on your digestive system. For example, a simple dish with chicken, bell peppers, olive oil, salt, and pepper is less likely to cause digestive upset than a more complicated recipe. **Bonus tip:** red bell peppers are often better for managing IBS than green and yellow bell peppers. This is because red bell peppers are fully ripened, which makes them easier to digest. When you buy fresh vegetables like mushrooms and bell peppers in bulk, it is convenient to freeze them later. This saves time and reduces the need for frequent shopping trips. Simply chop the vegetables, freeze them, and then use them whenever you are ready to cook. It is a simple way to manage your time efficiently and always have ingredients on hand for delicious meals.

By focusing on fewer ingredients, you can more easily identify and eliminate foods that might be challenging, helping to maintain a calm and balanced gut. Cooking simple meals can reduce stress during meal preparation and save time, which can positively affect overall digestive health.

Incorporating spices like black peppercorns into your meals can help manage IBS symptoms by aiding digestion and reducing inflammation in the gut. These spices contain compounds that promote the production of digestive enzymes, which can ease bloating and discomfort. They add flavour to dishes without excess salt or fat, making them a healthier option for those with IBS. Experimenting with different quantities of spices allows you to find the right balance for your taste preferences and digestive needs. So, do not be afraid to spice up your meals to improve your gut health and enjoy flavourful dishes while managing your IBS symptoms.

Cinnamon contains cinnamaldehyde, a compound known for its anti-inflammatory properties. These properties can help calm the digestive system and reduce gut irritation. It has also been shown to have antimicrobial effects, which means it may help fight off harmful bacteria in the digestive tract. Cinnamon's natural sweetness also makes it a great alternative to adding sugar to foods and beverages, which can be complicated for some individuals with IBS. Therefore, incorporating cinnamon into your diet can be a flavourful and beneficial way to support digestive health.

Stress-relieving foods

Using food as a therapeutic balm for stress can significantly help with IBS management. Certain foods can reduce bloating and help you look and feel younger. For example, foods abundant in antioxidants, such as berries, leafy greens, and nuts, can fight inflammation and stress in your body. Probiotic-rich foods like yoghurt and kefir can improve gut health and reduce IBS symptoms. Foods rich in omega-3 fatty acids, such as salmon and chia seeds, contribute to youthful-looking skin and promote gut health. Did you know chia seeds have more omega-3 than salmon? You can manage stress, reduce bloating, and promote overall well-being by choosing the right foods.

IBS-friendly superfoods

Adding amla and moringa to your diet can help manage IBS symptoms due to their high fibre content, which aids digestion and regulates bowel movements. These superfoods are rich in antioxidants and anti-inflammatory properties, which can soothe the gut and reduce discomfort associated with IBS. Conversely, millets are easily digestible gluten-free complex carbohydrate grains that provide sustained energy and stabilise blood sugar levels, lowering the likelihood of IBS flare-ups. Together, these foods contribute to overall gut health and can relieve IBS symptoms like bloating, constipation, and abdominal pain.

Hydration and digestive comfort

Hydration and digestive comfort are key to managing IBS. Incorporating foods with high water content, like cucumber and coconut water, can help hydrate the body and soothe the digestive system. Limiting legumes can reduce gas issues. Tea made from cumin seeds and carom seeds act as natural digestive aids to relieve discomfort. Opting for unsweetened drinks over carbonated ones and choosing regular Coke occasionally over diet options can help manage sugar intake and potentially avoid disrupting the gut microbiome. Being mindful of chemical sweeteners' impact on increased sugar cravings and gut health can contribute to better overall digestive wellness. So, making these simple dietary adjustments and choices can support your gut health and manage IBS symptoms more effectively.

Balanced snack choices

Choosing fibre-rich snacks like horsegram, a protein-rich lentil, and incorporating sweet treats with natural sweeteners like raw honey, maple syrup, or coconut sugar in moderate amounts can be beneficial for managing IBS symptoms. These snacks provide sustained energy and promote healthy digestion without aggravating the gut. However, it is crucial to be mindful of individual tolerances to particular sweeteners, especially those with fructose or sucrose intolerance. Experimenting with different options and observing how your body responds can help tailor your snack choices to support your digestive health. Including high-fibre options like dates, figs, and lentil cakes in your snacks can further aid in regulating bowel movements and promoting gut health. Figs contain fructose that those with IBS might not absorb well, so they should be consumed in limited portions. Choose cracker and rice cakes that do not contain wheat, barley, onion, fructose, and garlic powder. **Remember**, finding the right balance of fibre sweetness that works for you is critical to managing IBS effectively. Just remember, like anything, it is wise to enjoy them in moderation.

Healthier snack options

Choose biscuits made with low fermentable carbohydrates like rice or oat flour and gluten-free options such as quinoa. Opt for minimal ingredients, avoid artificial additives, and ideally make it homemade. Pick biscuits without fructose, oligofructose, inulin, apple juice concentrate, honey, wheat or soya flour. Some snack bars might have dates high in fructose, so watch out for those. Even though dates are high in fibre, they might cause issues for some individuals with IBS. It is suitable to have them in small amounts or make your own snack bars without these ingredients if they trigger symptoms.

For snacks, changing your environment to remove unhealthy options from sight or not buying them can be more effective than relying solely on willpower.

Quick and nourishing snacks

Incorporating quick and versatile snacks like boiled chicken breast with minimal salt, a dash of cumin, and turmeric for anti-inflammatory properties, paired with fresh salad and pomegranate, and enhanced with fresh lemon juice for flavour and natural vitamin C benefits, can be a smart strategy for managing IBS. This balanced and nutrient-rich option provides essential proteins, antioxidants, and anti-inflammatory compounds, promoting digestive health and overall well-being. This simple yet effective approach provides a clean source of protein and offers variety and convenience. Using boiled chicken breast for both snacks and meals, such as pairing it with salad for dinner or incorporating it into a chicken or vegetable broth for lunch, saves time and effort while ensuring a nutritious and satisfying option. **Personal tip:** opting for homemade chicken broth ensures no synthetic ingredients, making it a gentle choice that is particularly advantageous for individuals with sensitive digestive systems, particularly those with IBS.

Choosing gluten-free corn products such as corn tortilla chips, corn taco shells, and popcorn can be a good move for handling IBS, especially if you are sensitive to gluten. Corn is naturally gluten-free and tends to be easier on the stomach for many, which can help prevent IBS symptoms like bloating and discomfort. Corn tortilla chips offer a satisfying crunch and can be used in various meals and snacks. Remember to watch your portions and not overdo it, as overeating anything, even corn products, could worsen digestive problems. **Personal tip:** blue corn chips are a tasty swap for regular corn chips. They have a unique flavour, a bit sweeter than regular chips. Blue corn is full of antioxidants, which could help reduce inflammation. Adding these chips to your diet can mix things up and might be suitable for managing IBS.

Mindful indulgences of chocolate and oily snacks

Opting for moderate sweet snacks like dark chocolate or peanut butter on rice puffs can be beneficial for managing IBS symptoms, especially for those sensitive to high sugar intake. These snacks provide a satisfying indulgence without causing spikes in blood sugar levels or exacerbating digestive discomfort. Adding low FODMAP candies and dark chocolate with fresh fruits can further satisfy cravings while avoiding triggers like spicy deep-fried oily snacks and chocolates with wheat, like Kit Kat or biscuits, like Twix.

It is wise to always check ingredient labels and avoid low-sugar chocolate that contains polyols and carbs. Being mindful of ingredients can help prevent potential triggers and maintain digestive comfort. You can enjoy sweet treats without compromising gut health by choosing snacks that are gentle on the digestive system and mindful of personal tolerances. You can enjoy milk chocolate as it is low in lactose in moderate amounts, around 30 grams per serving. **Key takeaway:** choose dark chocolate with a cocoa content of at least 70%. It is better for those with IBS because it has less sugar and dairy than chocolates with lower cocoa content.

Choose sweets that do not have sugar, fructose, polyols, or liquorice. Instead, go for ones with glucose and sucrose, as they are better absorbed by individuals with IBS. Avoid most sugar-free chewing gum and mints as they often contain polyols such as sorbitol, mannitol, and xylitol, which can be unsuitable for some. Sugar versions may also have fructose, which is not ideal for those with IBS. Instead, try chewing on up to two pieces of fresh cloves daily. Cloves can help improve oral health and freshen your breath naturally.

Nourishing nut options

Including these top 9 nuts in your diet can be a valuable source of dietary fibre, which is beneficial for digestive health and managing IBS symptoms. Almonds, pistachios, walnuts, cashews, peanuts, pecans, macadamia, brazil nuts, and hazelnuts. Nuts contain good nutrition, like protein, fat, fibre, and vitamins. Eating them with healthy foods can help your heart and your immune system. Nuts add a tasty crunch to your snacks or meals. Enjoy them, sprinkle them over fruits and vegetables, or even toss them in sauces for added flavour and texture. It is recommended to eat nuts without adding salt or sugar. Remember, they are high in calories, so eat them in small portions, about two tablespoons per meal.

Understanding the protein and fat content of various nuts can assist you in making informed decisions about your diet. Some peanut and nut butter have extra oils and sugars to make them taste better, but it is better to pick ones without these. Which nuts are lower in calories? Peanuts and pistachios have a bit less. Hazelnuts and almonds have less saturated fat compared to others. If you are thinking about the least healthy nut, macadamia nuts have the most calories, and Brazil nuts have the most bad fat. By being aware of these nutritional facts, you can make smart choices that support your IBS management.

Increasing fibre intake can aid in maintaining regular bowel movements and reduce bloating associated with IBS. Dates are a great source of fibre and can be easily incorporated into smoothies and beverages for added nutritional benefits. When consuming nuts, ensure fructose absorption, moderation, and gas that leads to flatulence and bloating are considered.

Tip: soaking a mix of fresh nuts overnight and blending them with fresh coconut, a handful of curry leaves, a pinch of rock salt and cumin powder, and water not only improves their taste but also aids digestion, boosting your overall fibre intake. Biotin in nuts promotes healthy hair, which is an added bonus. Avoiding quick protein bars with high sugar content is essential as they can worsen IBS symptoms. Instead, opt for whole food sources of fibre to support gut health.

Bonus tip: soaking all fresh nuts overnight and peeling almonds makes them easier to digest, which is very helpful for individuals with IBS. This process reduces phytates, which can impair the absorption of minerals such as iron, zinc, and calcium. Soaked and peeled almonds are more nutritious and easier on your stomach. The skin of almonds has tannins, which can block nutrient absorption and may irritate a sensitive stomach. Soaking almonds overnight and peeling them removes these tannins, making the nuts gentler in your digestive system. Soak almonds in room temperature water with a pinch of salt. This makes peeling easier and activates enzymes that help with digestion. After peeling, you can blend the almonds into a smooth paste. This paste can be added to smoothies or dairy-free yoghurts for a nutritious and stomach-friendly addition. Add peeled, soaked almonds to oatmeal and salads, or eat them as a snack. They are full of healthy fats and proteins, which can assist in maintaining stable blood sugar levels and reduce IBS flare-ups.

Wasabi-coated peas can be a tasty snack, but they must be eaten carefully if you have IBS because they can be spicy and harsh on those with sensitive digestive systems. Start with a small amount, like a handful and pair them with a soothing food like plain rice or yoghurt to help balance the spiciness and reduce the chance of irritation. Limit yourself to small portions throughout the day rather than eating a large amount at once. Look for wasabi-coated peas that are less spicy. Drink water while eating to help with digestion and ease any spiciness. One of my personal favourites is Amazon's 'Sunburst Snacks Crispy and Spicy Wasabi Coated Peas, Resealable and Recyclable Packaging, 1KG' that can be purchased click here or check the 'Additional Resources' chapter for the complete link.

Balancing soluble and insoluble fibres

Soluble and insoluble fibres are essential in managing IBS but have different benefits. Soluble fibre dissolves in water, creating a gel-like substance, which can help regulate digestion and prevent diarrhoea. Good IBS sources include gluten-free oats and carrots. Apples can be an IBS trigger for some. Insoluble fibre adds volume to stool and assists in preventing constipation. Examples include whole grains, nuts, and vegetables like broccoli. Like Brussels sprouts containing raffinose, broccoli is part of the cruciferous family. This complex sugar is not easily digested in the human stomach. Once raffinose reaches the large intestine, gut bacteria ferment it, producing gas as a by-product. So, consuming them in moderation or avoiding them is critical for those with IBS. Aim for about 25-30 grams of total fibre per day for adults, with a mix of soluble and insoluble fibres. For kids, the recommendation is around 10-20 grams, depending on their age and size. Start with smaller servings and slowly increase consumption to minimise gas and bloating.

By including a variety of fibre-rich foods in your meals, such as adding a handful of berries with cinnamon to your breakfast yoghurt, whole grains with lean meat and vegetables at lunch, and a serving of bone broth with vegetables for dinner, you can take control of your IBS symptoms. This balanced intake not only helps manage IBS symptoms but also provides more energy and overall digestive health. **Remember,** soluble fibre like certified gluten-free oats, psyllium husk, and ground flax seeds are particularly effective at providing a more sustained energy release. Sometimes, psyllium husk works initially but becomes less effective over time. In such cases, eating more vegetables and flax seeds has personally helped with my IBS-C in regulating bowel movements. Millets contain more insoluble fibre than soluble fibre. However, millets still provide a balanced mix of fibre types, which benefits overall digestive health.

Gentle seafood choices for IBS

Cutting down on seafood that may increase body heat, especially when eaten in large amounts, like prawns, crab, and cuttlefish, and opting for fish instead could help manage symptoms of IBS. Each person's experience with IBS can vary, so finding what works for you is critical to managing symptoms effectively. Based on body types discussed in the chapter 'Potential Impact of Body Types on IBS', everyone's triggers and reactions to certain seafood can vary. Fish tends to be lighter and easier to digest compared to shellfish, which may be more irritating to sensitive digestive systems. Fish is also rich in omega-3 fatty acids, which have anti-inflammatory properties and can support gut health. By making this dietary adjustment, individuals with IBS may experience less discomfort and inflammation in their digestive tract, promoting overall IBS symptom management.

Mindful cooking practices

Using excessive amounts of oil in cooking can sometimes intensify symptoms of IBS, leading to discomfort and bloating. Opting for alternative cooking methods, such as water or silicone baking trays, can help reduce the amount of oil used, making meals easier on the digestive system. It is wise to select options like extra-virgin olive oil or cold-pressed oils, such as sesame oil, which are less processed and may be gentler on the stomach. Use a mix of oils like sesame for a week, then switch to olive and other healthy oils. This way, you get different nutrients from each oil, which is good for your health. Plain oils are suitable, and polyunsaturated or monounsaturated oils are preferred. Also, a heavy-bottomed pan can help distribute heat evenly and prevent burning, ensuring your food cooks well without excess oil. Margarines, low-fat spreads, butter, ghee, lard, and suet are IBS-friendly fats and spreads when consumed mindfully.

All types of vinegar, including cider, red wine, white wine, rice wine, and balsamic, are suitable for IBS. However, limit balsamic vinegar to less than 1 tablespoon per day to avoid stomach irritation.

Adjusting your cooking routine can help manage IBS symptoms and promote better digestive health. Using oils like olive, coconut, and avocado in a heavy-bottomed pan is brilliant for cooking. These oils can withstand high temperatures without burning, and the heavy-bottomed pan spreads the heat evenly, so your food cooks just right without getting stuck to the pan. Including oils in your diet is essential for managing IBS because they help maintain regular bowel movements and support overall gut health. Oils such as olive oil, coconut oil, and avocado oil offer healthy fats that can calm the digestive system and diminish inflammation in the gut, playing a critical role in reducing symptoms of IBS. These oils can aid in absorbing fat-soluble vitamins and nutrients, promoting overall well-being.

Beneficial complex carbohydrates

Incorporating complex carbohydrates like millet, wild black rice, and couscous into your diet can be beneficial for managing IBS. Soaking and pressure-cooking wild black rice can make it easier to digest, especially for individuals with sensitive digestive systems like IBS. This process aids in breaking down complex carbohydrates. It reduces the presence of anti-nutrients, making the rice more gentle on the stomach. Using pressure cooking preserves the nutritional value of the rice while making it soft and easy to chew, enhancing it's digestibility further. Wild rice options provide a nutritious and gut-friendly alternative to traditional rice varieties. These complex carbohydrates grains are rich in fibre, which aids in regulating bowel movements and enhances overall digestive health. They provide sustained energy release, keeping you fuller for extended periods and preventing spikes in blood sugar levels. One delicious recipe is a millet salad with mixed vegetables, grilled fish, and a lemon vinaigrette dressing.

Other high-complex carb options include quinoa and whole grains. Experimenting with different grains can add variety to your meals while providing essential nutrients for gut health and ensuring it is gluten-free for IBS trigger management, such as avoiding wheat, barley, and rye. These should also be limited or avoided by individuals with IBS who are sensitive to gluten or FODMAPs. Gluten-free foods highest in complex carbohydrates are quinoa, brown rice, gluten-free oats, buckwheat and amaranth. **Bonus tip:** if you are feeling adventurous with your food, try savouring gluten-free oats by cooking them with carrots, curry leaves, turmeric, water, and salt.

Mixing a variety of these complex carb grains and seeds in moderation each day can help maintain optimal long-term gut health.

Balanced protein intake

Animal protein makes meal planning more accessible because it contains all the essential amino acids in one source. On the other hand, plant protein requires careful selection and preparation to ensure you get the full range of amino acids. Both types of protein can be included in a healthy IBS diet, but if you prefer to stick to vegetable protein, that is your choice. Eating a balanced mix of animal and vegetable proteins can help manage IBS. Animal proteins like chicken and fish are often easier to digest for those with IBS and provide all essential amino acids vital for body functions. Vegetable proteins, such as beans and lentils, can also be beneficial but must be adequately cooked with asafoetida to avoid digestive issues like gas. Including both types ensures you get various nutrients and helps maintain muscle and tissue health, which is pivotal for overall well-being.

Opting for wild or organic chicken instead of regular chicken can improve gut health, especially for those with IBS. Wild chicken typically eats a more natural diet, which means it may have more healthy nutrients and fewer harmful antibiotics and hormones. Since wild chickens roam and eat various foods like insects, plants, and seeds, they may have healthier gut bacteria, which can help with digestion and reduce inflammation. So, choosing wild chicken can be a fresh approach to supporting gut health and managing IBS symptoms.

Reducing carbohydrates and opting for proteins is a wise choice for managing IBS. Proteins are more easily digestible and less likely to cause bloating and gas than carbohydrates. High-carb foods, significantly those high in FODMAPs, can trigger IBS symptoms like cramping, bloating, and diarrhoea. **Tip:** by focusing on protein-rich foods like lean meats, fish, eggs, and plant-based proteins, you can reduce digestive discomfort and support overall gut health. Also, proteins help stabilise blood sugar levels and support muscle repair, adding more benefits beyond managing IBS. Boosting your protein intake can enhance feelings of fullness, helping you feel fuller for longer. This can prevent overeating and promote a healthier weight, which benefits your gut health and overall well-being.

When picking frozen or ready-to-cook foods like chicken nuggets, fish fillets coated with breadcrumbs, or tempura batter, ensure the breadcrumbs are gluten-free and do not contain hidden onion and garlic in flavoured and spiced varieties. Many sausages contain wheat, onion powder, or milk, so check the ingredients list carefully.

Probiotic-rich foods

Kefir, kombucha, tempeh, and plain yoghurt are excellent for managing IBS when consumed in moderation because they contain live bacteria, also known as probiotics. These probiotics aid in preserving a balanced and healthy gut flora, essential for effective digestion and reducing IBS symptoms like bloating and discomfort. These foods support digestion and boost the immune system by enhancing gut health. **Bonus tip:** opting for plain yoghurt rather than flavoured ones is essential, as flavoured yoghurts often contain added sugars that can trigger IBS symptoms. Incorporating these foods rich in probiotics into your diet can contribute to establishing a more robust and balanced digestive system, leading to fewer flare-ups and better overall gut health.

Smart sweet treats

To manage sweet cravings while dealing with IBS, consider having dark chocolate, nuts, and green tea. When enjoyed in moderation, dark chocolate can satisfy your craving for something sweet without causing IBS flare-ups. Nuts provide a satisfying crunch and healthy fats that can curb cravings by keeping you full longer. Try to avoid nuts with saturated fats, as discussed earlier. Green tea is an excellent addition because it helps digestion and calms the stomach. **Tip:** combine dark chocolate with a handful of nuts for a satisfying snack that balances sweetness with protein and healthy fats. Drinking green tea can help soothe your digestive system and reduce inflammation, making this combination an intelligent choice for managing IBS.

Diverse meal components

Personal tip: balancing various flavours and textures in every meal, including sweet, salty, umami, sour, bitter, mildly spicy, crunchy, and creamy, can offer numerous benefits for managing IBS. By incorporating these elements, you can decrease sudden cravings, aid digestion, and break the monotony of a limited diet. This approach reflects traditional meal preparation methods, often emphasising diverse tastes and textures for optimal enjoyment and nutrition. Maintaining moderation and calorie control while experimenting with different flavours and textures is essential. Seeking out time-saving recipes that deliver diverse tastes and textures can help you achieve this balance efficiently, promoting gut health.

Nourishing bone broths

Bone broth, often known as "boner broth," is a nutrient-rich option for managing IBS symptoms due to its gut-soothing properties. Chicken or lamb bones are usually considered the suitable options for managing IBS due to their mild flavour, ease of digestion, and gentle effect on individuals with digestive sensitivities. The collagen in chicken broth promotes the growth of beneficial bacteria in the gut, supporting an overall healthy microbiome. It's collagen, gelatine, amino acids, and minerals help repair the gut lining, reduce inflammation, and support digestion, making it gentle on those with a sensitive digestive system.

For vegetarians and vegans, fresh vegetable or mushroom broths offer similar benefits, providing vitamins, minerals, and antioxidants to support gut health. Adding ingredients like seaweed or miso paste enhances the vegetable broths' flavour and it's nutritional value. **Personal tip:** to avoid onion and garlic in bone broth because it is a high FODMAP IBS trigger, consider using alternative herbs and spices like ginger, lemongrass, cinnamon and bay leaves to add flavour. You can include vegetables such as carrots, celery, and parsley for added nutrients and depth of flavour. **Remember** to let the bone broth cool down before refrigerating it to allow any excess fat to solidify on the surface. This makes it easier to skim off the fat, resulting in a cleaner and lighter taste when consumed later. Fats and excess oils are not suitable for those with IBS significantly, as they can heighten symptoms such as bloating and discomfort. Evidence suggests regular bone or vegetable broth consumption can help reduce IBS symptoms such as bloating, gas, and pain and promote overall digestive wellness.

Zinc and B12 for IBS

Getting enough zinc and vitamin B12 is essential for managing IBS because they help keep your gut healthy. Zinc supports your immune system and helps heal any damage in your gut. In contrast, vitamin B12 helps your nerves work correctly and can regulate digestion. You can obtain zinc from oysters, beef, pumpkin seeds and vitamin B12 from fish, meat, and dairy products. Enough vitamin B12 can ease tiredness, weakness, and stomach problems linked to IBS. The top 5 gluten-free B12 sources are fortified cereals, nutritional yeast, plant-based milk, eggs, and seafood like salmon. Fortified foods have extra nutrients added to them, not naturally found.

Monitoring your nutrient levels through regular check-ups and blood tests is essential. If your levels are low, supplements can be beneficial. However, it is necessary to consult with a healthcare professional before beginning any new supplements to ensure they are appropriate for you and do not interact with your IBS or any medications you are currently taking.

Calcium choices for IBS

Adults between 19 and 64 years old require a daily intake of 700mg of calcium. Taking more than 1,500mg a day can cause stomach pain and diarrhoea, but taking up to 1,500mg daily is generally safe and unlikely to cause harm.

Calcium is essential for bones, teeth, heart, nerves, and muscles. It can help manage IBS symptoms by regulating muscle contractions in the gut and reducing cramping and discomfort. About 99% of the body's calcium is in the bones and teeth. A calcium deficiency can cause calcium loss from bones and teeth, leading to lower back pain, neck pain, cracking sounds, tooth decay, cavities, and weak bones. Other symptoms include tiredness, disturbed sleep, and difficulty concentrating. If untreated, the body extracts more calcium from the bones, leading to fewer muscle contractions, skin problems, and premenstrual symptoms.

Calcium deficiency can result from a diet lacking calcium, weak digestion causing malabsorption or consuming too much sugar and caffeine, which also hinders calcium absorption. While dairy milk is a common source of calcium, increasing lactose intolerance and hormonal injections in cows raise questions about its suitability.

Five excellent vegetarian sources of calcium include a pinch of edible limestone mixed in curd, sesame seeds, horse gram, ragi millet, and amaranth millet (rajgira). Amaranth millet is 3.75 times more nutritious in calcium than quinoa and cheaper in Asian supermarkets. It is also an excellent source of protein and fibre, making it great for bowel movements and a balanced diet, especially for those with IBS.

Finger millet, also known as Ragi, is a vital grain widely grown in various parts of India and Africa. Ragi has the highest calcium content of all millets. For tips on making simple and nutritious millet recipes, refer to the previous chapter, "Microbiome-Friendly Foods and Recipes," and the section below "Gluten-free Millets for IBS Management." You can also find more ideas on the "Skinny Recipes" YouTube channel.

Selecting effective herbs for IBS relief

Adding herbs like dill, basil, oregano, fennel, and peppermint to your meals can help with IBS and optimise your gut microbiome. These herbs have natural properties that calm your stomach, reduce inflammation, and ease discomfort. They also add a tasty flavour to your food without needing lots of salt or spices. Try sprinkling them on salads, soups, or smoothies for a delicious and soothing touch to your meals.

For soups, adding fresh mint, coriander, or celery to soups and smoothies can help soothe the stomach, which is beneficial for managing IBS. Mint leaves help soothe the digestive tract, reducing cramps and discomfort. Coriander can help decrease bloating and improve digestion. Celery, a high-FODMAP, is rich in fibre and water, aiding bowel movements and preventing constipation when consumed in moderation, say one-third of a medium stalk. When consumed excessively, it can provoke symptoms in individuals with IBS. Dill leaves can also be used as they have anti-inflammatory properties that help calm the digestive system.

For example, you can prepare a refreshing mint and cucumber soup to soothe your stomach. Alternatively, blend coriander and celery with carrots into a green smoothie for a digestive boost. Adding dill leaves to a vegetable broth can add flavour and help soothe an irritated stomach. These simple changes can significantly impact how you feel.

To make tea with herbs like dill, basil, oregano, acai, fennel, melissa (known as lemon balm and part of the mint family), rosemary and peppermint, boil water, then steep a tablespoon of dried herbs or a few fresh leaves in a teapot or heatproof mug. Let it steep for 5-10 minutes before straining and enjoying it with lemon or honey. For spearmint tea, follow a similar process using fresh or dried spearmint leaves, steeping them in hot water for a few minutes before straining. Spearmint tea offers a refreshing taste and potential digestive benefits, soothing those with IBS. With its calming effects, Melissa herb may aid digestion and offer relief from gastrointestinal discomfort, benefiting individuals with IBS.

Peppermint oil tablets or fresh mint tea contain menthol that can help with IBS stomach pain and bloating by calming the stomach muscles. It is suitable for bloating and feeling uncomfortable after eating. Peppermint oil is concentrated and usually comes in capsules, or you can put a little bit on your skin. It is powerful and can help ease stomach problems like bloating and pain. **Personal tip:** drinking mint tea can be a gentle and safer choice. Mint tea is usually peppermint tea, which has a robust and cooling taste with a bit of sweetness. It feels refreshing and smells like menthol. Peppermint tea is often studied more for helping with IBS symptoms. It is essential to pay attention to how your body reacts to it. Spearmint tea, however, is made from spearmint leaves. It has a milder taste than peppermint, with a sweeter flavour and less menthol smell. Both teas can help you feel relaxed and refreshed. Individuals can choose between them based on which flavour and smell they prefer.

Chamomile tea can also calm the stomach but in a different way. It helps with stomach cramps because it can reduce inflammation. Ginger aids digestion and reduces feelings of nausea. Turmeric can reduce gut inflammation and discomfort. Fennel seeds help relieve gas and bloating. Adding these herbs to your diet or supplements might help ease your IBS symptoms.

Optimal dairy and fruit consumption

Eating dairy and fruits on an empty stomach can be a hurdle for those managing IBS. Dairy can cause bloating and discomfort because it is difficult to digest without other foods to slow down the process. When eaten alone, fruits can ferment quickly in the stomach, leading to gas and bloating. To help manage IBS, eating dairy and fruits as part of a meal with other foods is better. This slows digestion and reduces the chance of discomfort. For example, adding fruits to a bowl of oatmeal or having cheese with whole-grain gluten-free crackers can help make these foods easier on the stomach. This balanced approach can help keep IBS symptoms under control while still enjoying a variety of foods.

Limit fresh fruit intake with IBS

For managing IBS, it is ideal to eat up to three portions of fruit a day, with one portion being about 80 grams or what might fit in the palm of your hand, as discussed in the earlier chapter. For example:

- One medium-sized fruit like a banana
- Two smaller fruits like a satsuma or plum
- One medium slice of melon
- A handful of blueberries, grapes, or cherries

Eating whole fruits rather than smoothies or juices is better for fibre intake, as blending can reduce the fibre content.

Whole fruits help maintain healthy digestion, which is especially important for managing IBS.

Packaged fruit juices often have apples, even if not mentioned, so check the ingredients label and added sugars that are not good for those with IBS. Avoid squash and cordials that contain sweeteners, as these are IBS-trigger ingredients. If you do not have another option, add water to the packaged fruit drink to make it last longer. Canned and dried fruits should be eaten very sparingly by most individuals with IBS after careful thought because they often contain additives and sweeteners that can trigger flare-ups. **Bonus tip:** when buying prepared fruit in snack pots, note that they are usually sold in portions more significant than 80g, or use your palm to measure them, as discussed earlier. It is better to spread out eating them throughout the day rather than having it all at once.

Adding protein supplements to fresh fruit smoothies can worsen constipation for those with IBS, so avoid them unless necessary and always listen to your gut's reaction. It is better to stick with whole fruits to support gut health. **Personal tip:** replace fresh fruit juices and smoothies with millet smoothies, like those made with jowar, also known as sorghum. Check out the YouTube channel "Skinny Recipes" for many smoothie recipes. She also offers meals and various ideas without dairy milk or artificial sweeteners for those with IBS symptoms. Choose what suits your gut health.

Fermented foods for IBS relief

Fermentation breaks down complex nutrients, making them easier to digest, benefiting individuals with sensitive stomachs. Fermented foods like idly, dosa batter or pancakes made the night before can help manage IBS. Idly is a soft, steamed cake made from fermented rice and millet or lentil batter. At the same time, dosa is a thin, crispy pancake made from the same batter and cooked on an iron griddle. These South Indian foods contain probiotics that support gut health. The fermentation process enhances their probiotic content, aiding digestion and promoting a healthy gut microbiome, potentially reducing symptoms of IBS. Including these foods in your diet may offer digestive benefits, particularly for those with sensitive gut or digestive issues like IBS.

For IBS, idly dosa batter made with lentils like urad dal, split yellow mung, red lentils, green dal, and millet is often recommended. Add rava to the dosa batter for extra crispiness. These naturally gluten-free lentils and millets are more accessible to digest and less likely to trigger digestive discomfort than other varieties. Soaking the lentils overnight before grinding them into a batter can further enhance their digestibility. These lentils naturally rise over time due to the action of beneficial bacteria. Avoiding raising agents like bicarbonate soda is highly recommended. **Bonus tip:** ENO is a powder that aids in fermentation because of its acidic nature, helping to create a light and fluffy dosa or idly batter. You could replace ENO with gluten-free bicarbonate soda or avoid rising agents altogether, as they could trigger bloating and cramps for those with IBS. Fenugreek seeds and flattened rice can make a light and fluffy batter without rising agents, which can often trigger bloating in individuals with IBS.

Probiotic-rich foods for gut health

Kimchi, or pickled amla in apple cider vinegar and salt, provides probiotics and aids digestion. Kanji, a fermented rice soup with chicken and ginger, stimulates digestion and acts as a prebiotic. Exploring more fermenting techniques can offer further options for incorporating fermented foods into your diet, promoting digestive wellness and overall gut health.

The gut microbiome, made up of beneficial bacteria, is vital in managing IBS symptoms. Fermented soy products like tempeh and miso are rich in protein and beneficial bacteria, which can help reduce flatulence or gas, a common issue for those with IBS. Lacto-fermenting vegetables at home, such as pickles, cucumbers, carrots, and mild chillies, provide probiotics that support gut health.

Kimchi and kombucha are also great options in moderation, as they undergo natural fermentation, ensuring the presence of live bacteria and yeast. In the fermentation process of kombucha, the yeast produces alcohol, and bacteria produce lactic acid. This dual fermentation process results in the characteristic tangy flavour of kombucha, which is very low in alcohol content.

Tip: regular consumption of these fermented foods helps to maintain a healthy gut microbiome and reduce IBS symptoms. Consistency and moderation are essential, so incorporating a variety of fermented vegetables into your daily diet can promote digestive wellness. Eating homemade pickled vegetables and fermented soy foods regularly can contribute to a happy gut with improved IBS symptom management.

Tip: natto is made from fermented soybeans. It contains a beneficial bacteria called Bacillus subtilis, which can help improve digestion and support gut health. For those who do not enjoy the taste of natto, mixing it with other flavourful ingredients like soy sauce, mustard, or scallion tops (if onions are an IBS trigger) can help mask its intense flavour. Add it to dishes like rice bowls or salads where its taste can be better integrated. Consuming natto a few times a week can provide its benefits without overwhelming your taste buds.

Gluten-free millets for IBS management

Depending on the type of millet, it is rich in micronutrients like magnesium, iron, calcium, B vitamins, and zinc. These nutrients are crucial for immunity, especially for individuals with IBS who face nutrient absorption and fatigue challenges. Millet is naturally gluten-free, making it suitable for individuals with gluten sensitivities or intolerances. It offers a diverse range of nutritious options for IBS management.

A few examples of millets include ragi, buckwheat, sorghum (jowar), foxtail millet, and pearl millet (bajra). Pearl millet contains the highest amount of insoluble fibre, which feeds and nourishes beneficial gut bacteria. Children under 6 can enjoy millet-based pizzas, noodles, and bread. At the same time, older individuals, from youth to adults, are encouraged to consume more fibre. These millets can be quickly cooked as a supplement to rice. They can also be consumed as porridge combined with yoghurt and sea salt.

Millets are considered an alkaline-forming food, which is often recommended for achieving optimal gut health. It's soothing alkaline properties help maintain a healthy pH balance, crucial for preventing illnesses like acidity and heartburn for those with IBS.

They also have a low glycemic index, meaning they slowly release glucose into the bloodstream, which helps maintain stable blood sugar levels. This gradual release of glucose also provides sustained energy, avoiding sudden spikes or drops. Also, millet promotes a feeling of fullness sooner. It assists in weight management by curbing appetite and reducing cravings, unlike simple carbohydrates such as rice and wheat. White foods, notably "bad carbs" such as sugar and foods made from white flour, are often blamed for contributing to the obesity epidemic. Swap them with gluten-free whole grains if you have gluten intolerances, and aim for dietary diversity by including millets. As part of a balanced diet, including millets as about 30% of your food intake is generally recommended. This guideline promotes variety in nutrition and aims to incorporate whole grains like millet alongside other food groups. Adjustments may be necessary based on individual dietary requirements and preferences, so consulting with a qualified dietitian or nutrition expert can provide personalised advice for your health goals.

Millets are packed with essential nutrients that support your immune system. It can also be consumed as a fermented food, offering probiotic benefits for gut health. Traditionally, millets were fermented in clay pot dishes with raw unripe mango and green chilli to provide a refreshing and gut-friendly option during hot weather. Properly fermenting and storing these foods, whether by sun drying or refrigeration, ensures you get the most out of their probiotic benefits. It is essential not to reheat fermented foods to preserve their probiotic properties, and enjoying them within a day of making them ensures they retain their nutritional value. Refrigeration halts fermentation and extends the shelf life of food.

Here are some ways millets can be incorporated into your daily diet:

- Millet roti is a flatbread made from pearl millet flour and is popular in India. Other millets-based dishes include upma, khichdi, pongal, kheer, and laddoo.
- Injera: a fermented flatbread made from teff flour, a type of millet enjoyed in Ethiopia.
- Millet congee: a comforting porridge made from millet grains, commonly eaten in China.
- Tuwo Shinkafa: a millet pudding-like dish from Nigeria, often served with soups and stews.
- Polenta is a dish historically made from millet or cornmeal, and it is popular in Italy as porridge and cakes.
- Bori bap: a traditional Korean porridge made from millet and barley.
- Atole: a warm, thick beverage from Mexico made from masa harina, sometimes including millet for added texture and flavour.
- Millet based cheeseballs, biscuits, and cookies.
- New products made from millet include milk, soups and other innovative offerings such as millet-based vegan ice cream.

Bonus tip: mixing ground flaxseed with gluten-free millet flours can help manage IBS symptoms. Flaxseed is rich in soluble fibre, which can ease constipation and is often linked to IBS. It also contains omega-3 fatty acids, which can reduce inflammation and soothe abdominal discomfort. Adding ground flaxseed to gluten-free millet recipes boosts nutrition and improves the taste and texture of baked goods. These simple tweaks can offer a delicious and gut-friendly option for those with IBS, providing relief and enjoyment.

Ideal milk, yoghurt and ice cream options for managing IBS symptoms

Individuals handle milk differently based on their body types. Look for milk that says:

- Lactose-free / dairy-free (for those with lactose intolerance or dairy sensitivity)
- Preferably organic/ non-GMO (free from synthetic additives and pesticides)
- Derived from natural food ingredients (without artificial flavours or additives)
- Containing minimal processed sugars and fillers, which supports a healthier gut microbiome

Interesting fact: many adults start losing the ability to digest dairy milk properly as they age, particularly after 5 years. This is because the body produces less lactase, the enzyme needed to digest lactose, and the sugar in milk. As a result, they may experience symptoms like bloating, gas, and diarrhoea after consuming dairy. The prevalence of lactose intolerance grows with age, affecting many adults globally.

The suitable milk choice for many individuals with IBS is lactose or dairy-free. This type of milk removes the sugar (lactose) in regular milk, which can cause problems for those sensitive to dairy. So, if you have IBS, choosing lactose-free or dairy-free milk could help you feel better.

Most plant-based milk has flavourings unlikely to trigger IBS symptoms. It is wise to choose original and unsweetened options. Almond, coconut, soy, oat, quinoa, and rice milk are some examples of lactose and dairy-free alternatives. Lactose-free milk is an excellent source of calcium. Plant-based alternatives often have added calcium, but organic plant-based varieties usually do not.

Choose milk products without fruit concentrate, apple juice, fructose, or inulin. Sweetened milk drinks might have unsuitable apple ingredients.

You can use cow, sheep, or goat milk if you tolerate lactose. Rice and oat milk are the least likely to cause IBS issues, while lactose-free semi-skim milk can also work for some individuals. Almond, hazelnut, or other nut milk might only suit some, and coconut milk can be more watery.

Oat milk, in particular, is praised for its smooth texture and slightly sweet taste, making it a favourite among many. The starch in oat milk can spike blood sugar levels, but the increase is usually less than regular dairy milk. Nut milk is ideal and the unsweetened oat milk can be a better choice for people trying to control their blood sugar.

If you tolerate lactose, Greek-style and natural yoghurts are suitable. If you have trouble absorbing lactose, limit yourself to 2 tablespoons per meal. For larger quantities, choose yoghurts without fruits that cause IBS triggers, such as fructose, oligofructose, inulin, or chicory root.

Most ice cream and frozen yoghurt are okay if you can handle lactose. If you have trouble digesting lactose, stick to just one scoop of lactose-free ice cream per serving. There is no limit on portion sizes for dairy-free alternatives, including ice lollies. Avoid dairy-free ice cream and ice lollies with ingredients like biscuit pieces, cookie dough, brownie chunks, honey, forbidden fruits, or certain sweeteners mentioned above for yoghurts, including glucose-fructose syrup. Most flavourings in ice cream and lollies do not typically trigger IBS symptoms. For sorbets, look for varieties made with low-trigger fruits, avoiding apples, pears, and watermelon. Opt for natural sweeteners and avoid artificial ones like sorbitol, mannitol, and high-fructose corn syrup, which can cause stomach discomfort.

Creamy textured beverages for IBS

I prefer unsweetened oat, rice, and coconut milk instead of regular dairy milk because they do not contain lactose, an IBS trigger for some. Sometimes, I add one or two teaspoons of condensed milk for a creamy and sweet flavour. I swap out white sugar for condensed dairy three times weekly when I drink tea. I have one or two cups of tea daily, sometimes green or matcha tea and other times black tea with condensed milk or oat milk for creaminess. On other days, I enjoy plain black tea with a bit of jaggery, a natural type of unrefined cane sugar, or black tea with ginger. I also drink green tea with fresh lemon to add variety and a natural immunity boost. I always check the ingredients to avoid triggers like fructose. This has really helped me manage my IBS-C symptoms because I mix up my drinks throughout the week, which is better for my gut health.

Using condensed milk in tea can make it taste more affluent. Still, it might not be suitable for everyone with IBS-C or watching their sugar intake because it has a lot of lactose, which some individuals' sensitive guts do not like. I have tried it out and found that using condensed milk in minimal amounts makes my drinks more enjoyable without causing any discomfort. It is a good idea to use natural sweeteners like stevia, honey, jaggery, or maple syrup in small amounts, along with lactose-free or plant-based milk options, to make your tea creamy without the issues that condensed milk might bring. It is about finding and sticking with what works for your body. Choosing unsweetened milk and sweeteners that are low in FODMAPs is a good idea.

Jaggery is an unrefined sugar with the highest natural nutrients. It is produced by boiling sugarcane juice or palm sap until it solidifies and has a high FODMAP.

It retains more of the natural molasses and minerals found in sugarcane, giving it a brown colour and a distinct, deeper flavour similar to dark chocolate used in beverages and foods.

The powdered form is convenient for measuring and mixing into recipes. At the same time, the chunks are often used for traditional methods of sweetening beverages or dishes.

Tolerance to jaggery can vary among individuals. Some with IBS may find that they tolerate jaggery well, while others may experience symptoms. It is wise to start with a small amount and monitor your body's response to determine if jaggery suits you.

Everything good has to be eaten in moderation, with a variety each day and a healthy lifestyle.

I avoid granulated white sugar because it is heavily processed and tastes sweet, like white or milk chocolate. It has equal amounts of fructose and glucose. Brown sugar is not much better. It is just white sugar with added molasses. It contains sucrose that is broken down into equal parts glucose and fructose. Consuming too much sugar can trigger IBS symptoms, so it is wise to avoid both types of granulated white and brown sugar if you are prone to IBS triggers. White or brown sugar intake is not beneficial for maintaining healthy gut flora in the long term.

Instead, I use unrefined jaggery as a sweetener in my tea or ragi porridge. While it contains high sucrose levels, making it a high-FODMAP food, it is a natural option that can be healthier when used in moderation. Some believe that jaggery may have prebiotic properties, which could help beneficial gut bacteria grow and thrive. You might see some sediments when using solid jaggery, but they are safe to strain. I prefer powdered jaggery because it is easier to use.

Stevia might be suitable for IBS, but it is crucial to check product labels thoroughly. Pure stevia is generally safe, but some products may contain additives like erythritol, which could worsen your IBS symptoms.

Sometimes, I treat myself to coffee or green tea with a bit of raw honey, but mostly, I use powdered jaggery in my coffee. I pay attention to how my body feels each week and adjust how often I drink coffee to keep it in moderation. For sweetness, I use raw honey, condensed milk, or jaggery in moderation, ensuring that I spread the consumption of these items evenly throughout the week. Sometimes, I skip added sweeteners to give my system a break. This helps me manage my digestive health and maintain balance in my diet.

I use lists or an e-timetable on my phone to keep track of milk and sweetener choices, especially on days when I am more likely to experience IBS triggers. By paying close attention to how my body reacts to ingredients like jaggery, raw honey, and condensed milk, I have found it easier to manage digestive discomfort. This helps reduce fermentable carbohydrates (FODMAPs) in my diet, which can cause bloating, gas, and other digestive issues. Avoiding heavily processed low-FODMAP sweeteners like white and brown sugar is critical for gut health.

Most mornings, I enjoy plain matcha tea without sweeteners for a healthier gut. I use an electric milk frother to make it smooth and foamy, which helps me feel great for the rest of the day. Starting the day with smooth matcha tea helps me feel great without worrying about how it might affect my mood and performance later on. Experimenting with frothing has been fun. I can make silky lattes, foamy cappuccinos, and smooth Americanos. I bring green tea bags when I am out or travelling, as many cafes provide hot water.

Remember, it is crucial to listen to your body. Choose what works for your digestive health and personal tastes. If you are unsure how milk or sweetener alternatives affect your IBS-C symptoms, take it slow and consider consulting with a healthcare professional or dietitian for personalised advice.

Tips with beverages: trying different ways of frothing milk, drinking matcha and green tea, and exploring low-FODMAP unsweetened milk alternatives have helped me with IBS-C. If dairy milk causes IBS symptoms, avoiding it is prudent. You can find suitable milk and sweetener options mentioned earlier. This method allows for a balanced and enjoyable experience while managing symptoms and promoting digestive health. Coconut water is another safe choice for IBS.

Try this instead: challenge yourself to limit sweeteners in your beverages to twice a week or cut them out entirely as you age to help maintain a healthy gut microbiome. This habit can also boost your self-control, which may lead to positive changes in other areas of your life as time goes on.

Honey choices for IBS

Choose honey based on low FODMAP content, rawness, local sourcing, digestion and symptom management, avoiding added sugars, fructose, and polyol sweeteners. The ranking from the most to least preferred for managing IBS could be:

1. Raw honey retains more natural enzymes and antioxidants because it is not processed. I opted for 'Forest Field Honey' from the Baltic Honey Shop Store on Amazon, available here. It is unpasteurised, unfiltered, and has no added sugar - just like nature intended.
2. Low FODMAP honey: types like manuka or clover honey may be easier on the stomach. However, how you react can vary, so seeing what works for you is good.
3. Local honey: some think it might help with allergies and immunity because it contains local pollen. However, more proof is needed for this claim.
4. Plain, unflavoured honey: other honey might have added ingredients or additives that could trigger IBS symptoms. It is safer to stick with plain, unflavoured varieties.

Summary: even though honey is a natural sweetener, it still contains sugars that may ferment in the gut and contribute to symptoms in some individuals with IBS. Use honey in moderation and pay attention to portion sizes. I personally prefer raw honey.

The right honey for someone with IBS can differ from person to person. Pay attention to how your body reacts, and choose the honey that suits you by using it in moderation. Suppose you are still deciding which honey to pick. In that case, talking to a healthcare professional or a dietician is a good idea.

Selecting cheese and calcium intake for IBS

All cheese is suitable if you tolerate lactose. Most cheeses are low in lactose. Eat only up to 2 tablespoons per day of the following cheeses as they contain some lactose, such as processed cheese slices, reduced-fat cheddar, low-fat cream cheese, cottage cheese, ricotta, quark, or halloumi. Choose cheese that does not have forbidden fruits, onions, or garlic in them.

When managing IBS, you can replace cheese with lactose-free or low-lactose options to ease digestive discomfort. Aged cheeses like cheddar, swiss, or parmesan are naturally lower in lactose due to the ageing process and higher in protein. Non-dairy cheese alternatives such as nuts, soy, or coconut are suitable substitutes.

Some individuals may find goat or sheep cheese more straightforward to digest than dairy milk cheese and may contain less lactose. Opt for firmer cheese varieties like gouda, edam, parmesan, feta, mozzarella or manchego, as they tend to have lower lactose content than softer cheeses like brie, cream cheese, camembert and goat.

Aim for 700 mg of calcium daily for adults, essential for healthy bones and teeth. Have 2 to 3 servings of calcium-rich foods daily, like cheese, yoghurt, canned fish with edible bones, tofu, filtered tap and mineral water, calcium-enriched oats and other foods to ensure enough calcium. Organic varieties usually do not have added calcium. Aim to consume 2 to 3 portions of milk alternatives daily, such as one 200 ml glass of milk, one small 125-150 g pot of yoghurt, or 30 g of cheese, which is about the size of a small matchbox as discussed in earlier under 'Use your palm to gauge portion sizes' section.

Experimenting and finding the ideal options that suit your tolerance and preferences is essential. Check the nutrition labels for lactose content, consume cheese in moderation, and monitor how your body responds to ensure it does not amplify IBS symptoms.

Monitoring salt intake

Check food labels for low salt content to combat salt-related IBS flare-ups when shopping. Aim for less than 2000 mg/day of salt for adults, equivalent to less than 5 g/day, just under a teaspoon. For children aged 2–15 years, the study recommends adjusting the adult salt intake downward based on their energy requirements. Ensure all salt consumed is iodised for iodine intake. **Personal tip:** using sea rock salt over regular table salt offers more minerals such as magnesium, potassium, and calcium, which can positively affect overall gut function.

Choosing low-salt products

Opt for fresh, minimally processed foods in your diet. Look for low-salt products containing less than 120 mg of sodium per 100 grams. The Fooducate app, a free nutrition scanner, provides detailed insights into scanned foods, including ingredients and nutrient composition. With the ability to scan over 250,000 product barcodes, it simplifies shopping and empowers informed dietary decisions. Cooking with minimal or no added salt, relying on herbs and spices for flavour, and avoiding excessive use of commercial sauces can make a significant difference. **Bonus tip:** seaweed flakes, containing natural glutamates, enhance the umami flavour in foods, making them a flavourful alternative to salt.

Check the sauce label for salt and oil content

Aim for sauces with low salt content (less than 120 mg of sodium per 100 grams) and minimal added oils. Carefully reading sauce labels can help you make better choices. Look for:

- Low-sodium options include choosing sauces labelled as "low-sodium" or "no added salt."
- Healthy oils: prefer sauces made with healthy oils like olive oil, and avoid those with trans fats or hydrogenated oils.
- Minimal ingredients by selecting sauces with a short ingredient list and avoiding artificial additives or preservatives.

Sauces made with natural ingredients can also introduce beneficial antioxidants and anti-inflammatory properties into your diet. This helps manage IBS symptoms, supports overall gut health, and boosts your immune system. Making these mindful choices can enhance the flavour of your meals, making healthy eating more enjoyable. Choosing sauces with lower salt and oil content can help reduce IBS triggers while supporting better digestive health.

Italian sauces, salad dressings, and pesto usually contain onions and garlic, which can upset some with IBS. Instead, try tomato sauces with basil and oregano with gluten-free, wheat-free, and soy-free pasta. Make your pesto with basil, pine nuts, olive oil, and parmesan cheese, and skip the garlic. You can also try red pepper or basil pesto with chives for flavour without causing IBS symptoms.

The safest, IBS-friendly salad dressings are made by mixing lemon or lime juice with vinegar, olive oil, chopped mint, parsley, coriander, and a pinch of salt and pepper. Store this mix in a jar for 2 to 3 days. You can add tabasco sauce, mustard, a little chilli, crumbled feta, or blue cheese for more flavour.

Many sauces, like brown sauce and barbecue sauce, contain ingredients like apple, fructose, glucose-fructose syrup, onion, garlic, honey, and lactose milk in mayonnaise, which can trigger symptoms for those with IBS. These sauces may also include flavourings that could be derived from onions and garlic, making them unsuitable. Have them in moderation or eliminate them based on your trigger symptoms.

Oyster sauce is usually gluten-free, but it can sometimes not be, while traditional soy sauce contains gluten. Always choose gluten-free sauces and check the labels. **Key takeaway:** be bold about carrying your own sauces in small bottles. IBS bloating and discomfort can last for days or weeks, so it is vital to have safe options.

Thai and Chinese ready sauces often have onion and garlic, which can be bad for worsening IBS. Instead, try plain rice noodles. Enhance the flavour with fresh herbs, dried herbs, and various spices. Adjust the flavours to your liking to prevent cravings after your meal to make a sauce that is not too spicy, sweet, or sour. Aim for a balanced mix of flavours in your meal to help reduce cravings afterwards. Another option is asafoetida powder, or hing, a spice used in Indian cooking. It has an onion-like flavour and gets milder when cooked in oil. Try using infused oils like garlic, chilli, or herb for flavour without making it too spicy.

Baking with gluten-dairy-wheat-nut free ingredients

When baking gluten-free cakes, choose gluten-free baking soda instead of ENO. If preferred, swap butter for a dairy-free spread. Mix dairy-free spread with icing sugar, vanilla, and cocoa powder for a simple icing idea. Use more dark chocolate for cake toppings and cocoa nibs instead of chocolate chips for cookies to reduce sugar content and enjoy a guilt-free treat that supports your digestive health. Cocoa nibs offer an intense chocolate flavour without added sugars. Creative Nature's website offers IBS-friendly products and recipes with allergens clearly listed.

When dining out and craving cake, opt for ones without fruits known to trigger IBS, like apples, pears, wheat, or added fructose. Choose simpler cakes to avoid digestive problems. You can also make your own wheat-free cake.

My personal favourites include the Gluten-Dairy-Wheat-Nut-Free Carrot Cake and Banana Cake mix. They are super quick, soft, and moist, rise up well, delicious without doubt, and free from IBS triggers. You can find more similar products at creativenaturesuperfoods.co.uk. Use the discount code **JANN20 to** get 20% off everything. They also offer global shipping to around 18 countries, including the UK, USA,

Canada, Europe, Australia, UAE, and Singapore. Check out their website and click here for quick, easy, IBS-friendly recipes.

Wheat-free baking flour alternatives include arrowroot, chestnut, corn, potato, rice, cassava, plantain, teff, sorghum, fonio, and tapioca flour, to name a few. Naturally, gluten-free millet flours like sorghum, finger millet known as ragi, and pearl millet flours are great for baking because they can rise well and give baked goods an elastic texture. You can also use commercial gluten-free flour mixes for baking. Other helpful ingredients for wheat-free baking are ground almonds, gluten-free baking powder, buckwheat flour, cornmeal, ground hazelnuts, and Xanthan gum. Use nuts in moderation, up to 25g per portion, and mix them with other gluten-free flours to achieve balanced texture and flavour, as well as elasticity and the crumb texture in your baking.

Golden syrup is generally a better option for individuals with IBS than high-fructose sweeteners like honey. However, use it in moderation because too much of any sweetener can cause digestive discomfort. Always listen to your body's response and adjust as needed.

Healthier fast food choices

For individuals with IBS, choose grilled meals over fried options. For IBS-C, consider baked or air-fried potato wedges flavoured with herbs and spices for a healthier alternative to traditional deep-fried French fries. These contain less fat and are less likely to worsen symptoms. Most crisps and savoury snacks, mainly plain or salt and vinegar flavours, are usually safe to eat. However, be careful because some might contain onion or garlic, even if not mentioned in the description. **Bonus tip:** use a small bowl to portion out crisps, including healthier options like popcorn to avoid overeating. Portion management is critical for IBS symptom management. If you see ingredients like "maltitol" or "molasses," those might not be suitable, or you should only have a small amount, like one teaspoon per meal. So, check the ingredients list to make sure they are okay for you to eat.

Tip: consider replacing deep-fried foods with crispy alternatives like roasted vegetables or baked chickpeas. However, individuals with IBS may discover that high-fibre foods such as chickpeas are challenging to digest and can lead to increased gas. **Try this instead:** soak chickpeas overnight before dry roasting or baking. This helps reduce gas production by discarding the soaking water and using fresh water for cooking. Adding asafoetida, a spice that aids digestion and adds flavour while reducing gas, can also be beneficial. Removing the chickpea skins may make them easier to digest for some individuals.

Grilled or baked turkey or chicken burgers served on a whole-grain, gluten-free bun or lettuce wrap can be a suitable substitute for traditional beef burgers, as they are typically lower in fat and easier to digest.

Choosing low-fat, low-sodium chicken or turkey sausages without added preservatives or spicy seasonings can be a good alternative. These sausages are usually more accessible to the digestive system than traditional pork sausages because they contain less fat. Lower fat content can help reduce symptoms of IBS, such as bloating and constipation, making them a milder choice for individuals with sensitive digestive systems.

Suitable pizza alternatives

A suitable substitute for pizza could be a homemade version using a whole grain or gluten-free crust, low-fat cheese, and a variety of cooked vegetables like bell peppers, mushrooms, and spinach. Limiting high-fat toppings like pepperoni and opting for a lighter tomato sauce with less oil in the sauce mix can also help reduce the risk of triggering IBS symptoms. Check the sauce label for salt and oil content.

Bonus tip: eating junk food, such as pizza, can worsen bloating for those with IBS. This happens because junk food often has lots of salt, which makes the body hold onto water, causing bloating. However, there is a clever twist! Drinking water with these healthier pizza options, which have less salt and fat, can further help reduce bloating. Good fats need to be eaten in moderation, too, to manage IBS well. Water helps flush out extra salt from your body, easing bloating. So, if you are craving pizza or junk food, **remember** to drink lots of water. This simple trick helps with managing IBS symptoms. Checking food labels to avoid high-salt and oil options or making special requests at restaurants and takeaways, can make a big difference in how you feel after eating. **Important fact:** what you eat today affects your gut microbiome immediately, hence the trigger symptoms we often face, which can impact IBS symptoms over time, affecting all areas of your life. So, it is wise to be mindful of your meals each day and nurture a healthy gut for the long term. This can help avoid needing medications later in life.

Adding Coke Zero or regular soda with occasional biryani

Adding Coke Zero or regular soda to your diet, especially when paired with indulgent Indian dishes like biryani consumed sparingly, can help manage IBS symptoms. Despite its delicious taste, biryani often includes spices and oily ingredients, which may not sit well with sensitive digestive systems due to their intense flavours. Having it rarely, like once every two months, gives your digestive system a break from potentially irritating foods.

Regular Coke has sugar, which can cause bloating and discomfort for some with IBS. Coke Zero has no sugar, but artificial sweeteners like aspartame might still be bothersome. Listen to your body to see which one suits you. Some find avoiding carbonated drinks helps, while others can have them in small amounts. It is about finding what feels good for you.

Remember to savour biryani occasionally and on its own. When you do indulge, accompany it with drinks that are gentle on your stomach, such as non-carbonated fresh juices with no added sugars or preservatives like lemon, pineapple, cranberry, grape, and orange juices. These options support better digestion and minimise IBS triggers, allowing you to enjoy a variety of flavours in moderation. **Tip:** drinking cranberry juice can help with IBS symptoms. It has antioxidants and anti-inflammatory properties that soothe inflammation in the gut, soothing any digestive discomfort that might arise from enjoying spicy or rich foods like biryani. Cranberry juice is full of fibre, which helps with regular bowel movements and relieves constipation. Make sure to choose pure cranberry juice without added sugars or artificial ingredients. Including cranberry juice as part of your diet can refresh and support your gut health. Try pairing room-temperature cranberry juice with your occasional biryani. Drinking icy beverages can slow down how quickly your body digests food. It is not just the ice that matters, but also how much cold food and drinks you consume. It is ideal to avoid having too many icy beverages, especially when having heavy foods like biryani. Making small changes to your drinks can help improve your digestion.

Being mindful with every meal while managing IBS is crucial for symptom management and maintaining optimal gut microbiome health. Paying attention to what you eat can identify triggers, make informed choices, and support a healthy balance of gut bacteria. This approach can significantly improve IBS symptoms and contribute to long-term digestive wellness.

Choosing gluten-free noodles for IBS relief

Picking gluten-free noodles for takeaway helps with managing IBS. Gluten, found in regular noodles, can often trigger uncomfortable symptoms like bloating and gas for those with IBS. However, gluten-free noodles, made from ingredients like rice or quinoa, are easier on the stomach and less likely to cause issues. So, next time you are ordering takeaway noodles, going gluten-free could make a big difference in how you feel afterwards.

Zucchini noodles are crafted from zucchini, a vegetable low in FODMAPs, making it an excellent choice for those with IBS. Other vegetables can also be spiralised to create noodles like zucchini noodles. These include carrots, sweet potatoes, butternut squash, cucumber, beetroot, turnips, parsnips, and daikon radish. Using these vegetables, you can enjoy delicious noodle alternatives that are both nutritious and gentle on the digestive tract, making them ideal for managing IBS.

Garlic and onion alternatives

Garlic and onions can make food tasty, but they contain fructans, which can mainly upset your stomach as it is not fully absorbed in the small intestine. If you have IBS. They might cause gas, cramps, and discomfort, even when cooked. This might include garlic and onion in the form of dried extract, powder, puree, and salt. They may be listed as "flavour," "flavouring," "natural flavour," or "natural flavouring." These ingredients are commonly found in stocks, stock cubes, and flavoured crisps, for example, and should be avoided. They are high-trigger foods for some individuals.

Luckily, there are alternatives. Horseradish, ginger, and asafoetida can give dishes a similar kick without tummy trouble. Asafoetida powder, also known as hing, is potent, so a sprinkle is enough to add intense flavour to dishes.

Garlic-infused oil with garlic pieces removed, scallions, chives, fennel, bell pepper, and leek leaves can add flavour without the FODMAPs when consumed in moderation. Use chilli oil in moderation, as it can be too spicy.

Fresh garlic scapes are usually better for those with IBS than garlic scape powder. The powder is milder than regular garlic powder. It is made from the green parts of garlic plants and is low in FODMAPs, which is good for IBS. However, it can still upset those with sensitive digestive systems because it has some compounds that might cause bloating. Some individuals might be fine consuming it in certain dishes, but it is safer to be careful. Fresh garlic scapes are often safer and can be a tasty addition to soups, dips and pesto, mashed potatoes, rubs, and salad dressings without causing as many issues. Consume fresh garlic scapes in moderation.

Shallots, radishes, fennel bulbs, and celery are some onion substitutes that add crunch to your salads.

Garlic-free seasoning shakes are blends of herbs and spices that add flavour to food without using garlic. They are great for those with IBS who need to avoid garlic triggers that can cause discomfort in the stomach.

Onion-free stuffing is made without onions, often including ingredients like herbs, celery, carrots, and gluten-free bread. These ingredients provide flavour and texture without the garlic and onion triggers.

Pick stuffing and all items without wheat or other gluten; avoid onion or garlic. You can try cornflakes, polenta, oats, or make your own breadcrumbs using gluten-free bread. The same goes for batter, pancake, and Yorkshire pudding mixes. Bread made from gluten-free oat flour, plain flour, or gluten-free self-raising flour is essential. Avoid soya flour, gram flour, chickpea flour, pea flour in your bread or all other baking flour mixes. Choose mixes without wheat, honey, and garlic. For stuffing, avoid store-bought mixes with onion and garlic in any form if sensitive. Instead, make your own with leftover bread or chestnut puree. Use chives or garlic scapes instead of onions for flavour.

To replace onions in chutney bases like Sri Lankan sambol and Indian onion chutney, you can try using shallots or asafoetida for a similar taste. Ingredients like tomatoes, bell peppers, or grated coconut add texture and flavour to your chutneys. Relishes and chutneys sometimes have ingredients like onion, apple, cauliflower, garlic, plum, or apricot, which can be high triggers for IBS if eaten in large amounts. Mango, another common ingredient in chutneys, should be avoided if you have fructose malabsorption. Instead, you can make homemade relishes or chutneys using suitable vegetables that are safer for digestion. **Key takeaway:** when choosing condiments, pick products that do not contain onion, garlic, apple juice, glucose-fructose syrup, or fructose.

New products are constantly being introduced, so it is important to explore them carefully to identify triggers and eliminate them where required based on your IBS trigger symptoms to maintain a healthy gut flora. Experimenting with these substitutes can enable you to enjoy delicious, varied, simple meals without experiencing IBS symptoms.

IBS-friendly curry and dessert thickeners

For gluten-free curry thickeners, you can use arrowroot, corn flour, or cream of tartar. In moderation, try mashed potato, greek yoghurt, heavy cream, or coconut cream for more curry thickeners. Adding cashew puree to curries makes them creamy, rich, tasty, and suitable for those with IBS. Also, dry roast and grind raw rice into a powder, adding it towards the end for a thicker curry consistency. If you are steering clear of onions and garlic to avoid thickening your curry, consider the alternatives we have talked about before in the garlic and onion alternatives section.

IBS-friendly dessert thickeners include agar-agar, cornstarch, arrowroot, tapioca, potato starch, psyllium husk powder, flaxseed meal, or mashed bananas. Ensure the custard powder is made up of lactose-free or nut milk.

Managing the costs of gluten-free food

Use less gluten-free bread and try millet, rice cereals, gluten-free oats, rice crackers, potatoes, rice, quinoa, wheat-free pasta, and rice noodles, which are usually cheaper. Naturally, gluten-free foods like millets, potatoes, rice, and quinoa are good options.

Freeze slices of wheat-free or gluten-free bread to prolong their shelf life and avoid waste. Purchase supermarket-brand bread, pasta, and other foods. Pay attention, as sometimes only well-known quality brands are IBS-safe, especially in the case of bread.

Purchase wheat-free flour in bulk and opt for supermarket brands, which are more affordable than well-known brands.

Bake your own wheat-free snacks like flapjacks and cakes. Select trusted brands like Creative Nature, and use the discount code **JANN20** when purchasing online to get 20% off all their products. They ship to 18 countries, providing access to safe and dependable IBS-friendly products and recipes.

Choose seasonal and cheaper vegetables like carrots, courgettes, green beans, and potatoes.

Buy frozen fruits like raspberries and vegetables like spinach, okra, and green beans.

For milk alternatives, pick supermarket-brand lactose-free or nut-free milk.

Low-salt, gluten-free sauces and ready-made meals can be convenient yet expensive. Cooking at home in bulk or frequently, especially if you prefer using fresh ingredients, is often more economical.

Look for cheaper food options in the cooking aisle compared to the whole foods aisle at supermarkets.

The above tips and reading food labels ensure that IBS-friendly foods are affordable and manageable.

Food combinations to avoid for IBS management

Food Combinations	Reason
High-fat and spicy foods	Irritate the digestive system, leading to bloating and discomfort
High-fibre foods with large meals	Overwhelm the digestive system, causing gas and bloating
Dairy and high-fibre foods	Difficult to digest for some, leading to digestive discomfort
Alcohol and carbonated beverages	Irritate the gut lining, worsening symptoms like bloating and gas
Raw fruits and vegetables	Hard to digest especially in large quantities or on an empty stomach

Self-created table by Jan Nallathamby content from PubMed Central

The above table highlights the importance of having small portions of different flavours and nutrients instead of overindulging in one type of food, which can trigger IBS symptoms and discomfort. This approach requires careful meal planning and minor, mindful tweaks to your diet daily. Practising this consistently can lead to long-term benefits and improved well-being by promoting a happy gut.

Planning your meals and snacks in advance, say 1-2 weeks, especially for meals away from home, can enable you to enjoy a broader range of foods, avoid wrong food combinations and stick to your IBS-friendly diet more efficiently. Always seek personalised dietary advice from your doctor.

CHAPTER RECAP:

Meal planning can significantly help manage IBS symptoms, though it might not solve everything immediately. IBS is a functional disorder, so symptoms might not disappear completely. It requires consistent effort, along with stress and exercise management, daily.

Most foods contain FODMAPs, which many individuals do not absorb well. Still, those without IBS usually do not feel any symptoms. Only restrict FODMAPs if they make your IBS worse. They are in many foods, even healthy choices, but only cut them out if they are very high IBS triggers such as onion and garlic or have tiny portions of medium or low trigger foods, say once in three days or once a week if you experience IBS symptoms. Experiment with your food; occasionally reintroduce high or medium-trigger foods and remove them to see how your body reacts.

For many with IBS, certain foods and drinks containing fructans, such as sugar snaps, pears, and figs, galactooligosaccharides (GOS) found in beans and pulses that cause wind or flatulence, polyols such as sorbitol and mannitol found in coconut and cauliflower, along with lactose, are the main triggers of symptoms. Lactose in small amounts is usually tolerated well by most with IBS, but try to avoid sorbitol and mannitol added as binders or fillers.

Bonus tip: refer to the food chart nutrition guide for the IBS meal plan and gut health trackers mentioned earlier for additional foods containing these triggers. To maintain a healthy microbiome, it is wise to consume them in tiny amounts less often, say every three days or once a week, along with a varied, balanced diet every day that causes no IBS triggers for you. Add different colours of food and drinks to your diet for more variety. This takes patience and lots of trial and error. Your choices may change depending on your stress levels, hormones, location, and other factors. Personalise your food and beverages since the personal tolerance threshold varies. If I can do it, so can you.

Avoid using dietary enzymes like lactase tablets or drops that digest lactose, as these products may contain sorbitol or mannitol. They are usually required when trigger foods are eaten in large amounts. Avoiding all enzymes and managing your food intake for a healthier gut is prudent. Many consider Hippocrates, the father of modern medicine, to have said, "Let food be thy medicine and medicine be thy food."

The "free from" section in supermarkets is perfect for finding IBS-friendly food, especially if you are sensitive to many IBS-trigger foods. Gluten-free, starchy foods are typically safe to eat for most individuals. Still, it is essential to check for other ingredients that could be triggers for IBS, like apple, date paste, dried fruit, fructose, honey, milk, inulin, oligofructose, FOS, garlic, onion, and sorbitol if there are your trigger ingredients. Consult a dietician for further help.

Choosing foods mindfully and sticking to natural, diverse options, such as fresh, pickled, fermented, sprouted, and fibre-rich foods and various immunity-boosting foods with multiple vitamins and minerals can help control your symptoms and improve overall well-being. Pay attention to your body and avoid triggers that worsen your symptoms. Focus on a low-FODMAP yet varied diet for long-term success, eliminating only the very high IBS trigger foods. This varies from person to person and can be done using techniques such as journaling, symptom tracking, healthy routine habits, and meal planning tips discussed above. **Key takeaway:** getting addicted to any food or drink, like coffee, alcohol, biryani, or even addiction to healthy options can be harmful. Having too much of anything, whether good or bad, can harm your health. The unhealthy addictions provide quick dopamine boosts, which is a brain pleasure chemical and can lead to more cravings. Training your taste buds to enjoy diverse foods and drinks is essential. This helps manage IBS better and keeps you healthier overall.

Understanding visceral hypersensitivity is important because high-FODMAP foods can cause gas, leading to pressure and false alarms in your brain. This can cause distress, anxiety, diarrhoea, constipation, and pain. Techniques like hypnotherapy can also help calm the gut and reduce false alarms that trigger IBS symptoms.

When dealing with IBS, it is frustrating not knowing what triggers symptoms. Keeping a food diary can assist in monitoring your eating habits and their effects, reveal patterns, and identify challenging foods. During an IBS attack, stick to simple, easy-to-digest foods like bananas, rice, apple sauce, and toast (BRAT diet) to calm your stomach. Many with IBS find that apples can make their symptoms worse. So, it is a wise idea to steer clear of them if you are dealing with IBS. If you are feeling constipated, go for ripe bananas. They are gentle on your stomach and can help you clear your bowels easier. If you are dealing with a runny poop, opt for bananas that are a bit greenish-yellow. They are more starchy and can help make your poop firmer.

Listen to your body and adjust your diet, giving it time to heal between flare-ups. Discovering what works for you involves experimentation, which is necessary since triggers vary for each individual.

Eating a variety of leafy greens, fermented foods, and fibre-rich foods can help manage IBS symptoms. Along with a varied, balanced diet, it is safe to avoid medications unless you have other health conditions and stick to natural, diverse foods.

Consistent, mindful eating and stress management can improve gut health and overall well-being by reducing IBS flare-ups, flatulence, or wind. **Key takeaway:** be cautious about what you eat today, as it immediately affects your gut health. Be intentional with your food choices. Avoid complicated food combinations and carefully read labels. Pay attention to calorie and nutrient intake, meal diversity, and portion sizes for every meal. These are key for IBS trigger management. Everything you eat in each meal influences your mood, gut health, and performance quickly, ultimately impacting your gut microbiome in the long run. Consistently exploring different food options and cuisines provides both variety and balanced nutrition.

19. Stress Management Techniques for IBS Relief

"He who has health, has hope; and he who has hope, has everything." — Thomas Carlyle

Understanding good and bad stress is essential for managing IBS. Good stress, also known as eustress, can help with IBS by making you feel good and motivated. For example, regular exercise like yoga or walking helps relax your body and improve digestion. Learning new skills or hobbies can keep your mind busy and distract you from IBS discomfort. Spending time with friends and family, doing creative activities like painting or writing, and achieving work goals can lift your mood and reduce stress, leading to fewer IBS flare-ups.

Bad stress, also known as distress, can make IBS worse by increasing anxiety and tension. Stress from work pressure, financial problems, and relationship issues can keep you worried and stressed, which affects your digestion. Health worries and significant life changes, like moving or losing someone close, add emotional stress and can worsen IBS symptoms.

To manage IBS better, focus on creating good stress and reducing lousy stress. Try mindfulness or meditation to handle work stress, get financial advice to manage money worries, and build strong, supportive relationships. Understanding the contrast between positive and negative stress by focusing on positive activities can boost your digestive health and overall well-being.

Managing IBS can be challenging, but reducing stress and adopting simple habits can help. Stress can worsen IBS, so it is essential to find ways to relax. Stress-related IBS symptoms include abdominal pain, bloating, diarrhoea, constipation, and nausea.

Activities like taking long, sometimes short, consistent walks also help; reading, meditating, daily gratitude, mindfulness, praying, or taking a detox bath can be very beneficial. Keeping a record of your stress and IBS symptoms helps identify patterns and triggers using the trackers and journals mentioned earlier. You can use your phone's notes or calendar to jot down stressful events, your reactions, and how you plan to handle them better next time. Partake in mentally and physically comforting activities such as the below.

Introduce play with productivity

Make time for fun and relaxation every day. It has to be scheduled rather than a milestone celebration to manage stress effectively. Slowing down and enjoying work, exercise, and relationships can improve your mood and creativity. Learn from mistakes and find humour in them while connecting with your thoughts by tuning into your body through the 2-minute body scan meditation morning routine discussed earlier.

Every day, give yourself the freedom to step away from duties and to-do lists, embracing happiness and playfulness regardless of age, for long-term management of IBS. **Key takeaway:** regular downtime and scheduling daily play activities can boost focus and creativity in all aspects of life, making them ideal for managing IBS.

Move slowly and quickly throughout the day

Regular movement throughout the day is critical for managing IBS symptoms. Even a brief 20-minute walk, especially on busy days, can positively impact gut health and is better than no activity. Avoid prolonged sitting, as it can negatively affect gut health. **Tip:** keep moving. 'Sitting is the new smoking.'

Splitting your post-lunch 20-minute mandatory walk into a 10-minute brisk walk and a 10-minute light jog can greatly benefit IBS management. This approach not only helps with digestion but also prevents long periods of sitting, which can worsen gut health. I am vouch for its effectiveness. Including short bursts of movement throughout the day helps regulate bowel movements and reduces discomfort. Alternating between activities keeps your body and mind engaged, promoting overall well-being and productivity.

Staying active with gentle, regular movements every hour and frequent breaks is essential for managing IBS stress and productivity.

Establishing a calming bedtime routine and deep sleep

Developing a relaxing bedtime routine is crucial for effectively managing symptoms associated with IBS. Aim to sleep by 10 p.m. and get at least seven hours. Make your sleep environment comfortable, and practice relaxation techniques to improve sleep quality.

Reducing screen time, especially before bed, helps manage IBS, as excessive screen use can cause stress and eye strain. Implement a "digital curfew" an hour before bed. Aim for 30 minutes of 'digital curfew' or screen-free time before sleeping. Use this time for relaxing activities like reading or gentle yoga. This reduces blue light exposure, boosts melatonin production, and helps achieve deep sleep, essential for stress reduction and digestive health.

Including the 'pliability: mobility + recovery' app for stretches in your night routine can help with IBS. It relaxes your muscles and reduces tension in your stomach, which can ease IBS symptoms at night. The app guides you on the ideal stretches, ensuring you target the right muscles. This interactive and enjoyable app makes it easier to stick to your stress-free nighttime routine. This sets the stage for a brighter morning ahead. Doing these stretches regularly can create a calming habit that reduces IBS symptoms and makes you feel better overall.

After 10 p.m., you might feel a 'second wind' of energy that lasts until 1 a.m. This burst of energy is meant for organ cleansing, especially by the liver. To support your body's natural process, try to sleep before this second wind hits unless you work night shifts. Focus on getting deep sleep, about 20-25% of your total sleep, which is fundamental for physical and mental recovery.

Following your natural body cycles to improve sleep, manage stress, and support digestion. The liver detoxifies the body between 1 a.m. and 3 a.m., so deep sleep is crucial. For those with IBS, it is wise to avoid late-night activities and focus on a calming bedtime routine. This helps the liver's detoxification process and promotes overall gut health.

Spending time in nature and holistic care

Being in natural surroundings can reduce stress levels and enhance overall well-being, so spend time outdoors daily, whether for work or leisure. Firstly, spending time in nature helps you relax. When surrounded by trees, flowers, and fresh air, it calms your mind and body, reducing stress that can trigger IBS symptoms. Secondly, being outdoors encourages physical activity. Whether walking, jogging, or simply enjoying the scenery, moving your body can aid digestion, especially after meals for 20 minutes, which should do the trick and relieve discomfort associated with IBS. Thirdly, breathing in fresh air is good for your overall health and digestive system. It can help improve your well-being and ease digestive issues. Lastly, being in nature promotes a sense of connection. Feeling connected to the environment can encourage emotional balance, which can reduce the severity of IBS symptoms.

Incorporating simple breathing exercises around nature into your morning routine can promote calmness and reduce stress, as discussed earlier.

Taking care of your skin with cooling foods like amla, rich in vitamin C and fresh aloe vera drink, or through self-massage application onto the skin can help balance and cool the body. This holistic approach can benefit individuals with a dominant Pitta dosha, which can trigger IBS symptoms. Cooling foods and practices help reduce body heat, ease digestive issues and promote overall gut health. You can support better digestion and a calmer gut by including these natural methods in your routine.

Hobbies that reduce stress

Boxing is a fantastic stress management tool for IBS, as it helps release pent-up tension and promotes overall well-being for those with IBS. Other stress management daily hobbies include gardening, cycling, writing, photography, yoga, weight lifting, basic strength training, hiking, nature walks, drawing, painting, crafting, DIY projects, playing musical instruments, knitting, crocheting, singing, cooking, baking, and taking part in activities or hobbies that bring happiness and relaxation. **Bonus tip:** continuously explore new stress-relieving hobbies and content through podcasts, social media, and books. Maintaining a curious and open mind leads to ongoing self-learning and growth.

Tip: performing quantum-guided meditation with light language and high-frequency codes can start to remove obstacles in your body and mind, aiding in managing IBS. By blending ancient wisdom with modern techniques, it addresses physical and emotional issues associated with the condition. This innovative approach goes beyond IBS symptom management, targeting deeper emotional and energetic healing levels. Regularly practising this technique can lead to reduced stress and an improved sense of well-being, promoting holistic healing for individuals with IBS.

CHAPTER RECAP:

Managing IBS can be tricky, but there are simple habits that can help. Stress can worsen IBS, so finding ways to relax is essential. Activities like taking walks, reading, meditating, practising gratitude, and mindfulness can all be beneficial. Tracking stress and IBS symptoms helps identify patterns and triggers. Regular downtime and scheduled play activities can improve focus and creativity, which is essential for managing IBS. Adults often underestimate play, but it can be a real game-changer.

Moving throughout the day is crucial for managing IBS symptoms. Even brief walks can have a beneficial effect, so avoiding long periods of sitting is essential, especially in jockey jobs. Establishing a calming bedtime routine and ensuring deep sleep is vital for managing IBS symptoms. **Key takeaway:** using stress positively helps manage IBS well. Striking a balance between tension and relaxation allows your body to adapt and become stronger, building resilience. Each person's stress levels vary, and not all stress is harmful.

Spending time outdoors can help reduce stress and improve well-being, which benefits IBS management. Incorporating hobbies that reduce stress, like boxing or gardening, can also help. Quantum-guided meditation with light language and high-frequency codes can aid in managing IBS by addressing both physical and emotional challenges linked to the condition. These techniques provide holistic approaches to managing IBS stress symptoms, impacting gut health, mood, performance, and life fulfilment.

By regularly practising a balanced mix of these techniques each day, with a holistic mindset, you can effectively manage stress-related IBS symptoms such as abdominal pain, bloating, diarrhoea, constipation, and nausea.

20. Exercise and it's Impact on Gut Health

"The only time you run out of chances is when you stop taking them." — *Alexander Pope*

This chapter discusses how exercise affects gut health, focusing on how staying active helps digestion and managing IBS symptoms. It will also explain how maintaining a healthy BMI and weight through exercise can improve IBS symptoms. It explores some new and personalised exercises that can help keep your gut healthy while also making you feel better overall.

Exercise and the gut-brain connection

Being healthy and at peace truly makes us happy. Exercise can help our gut and IBS symptoms by connecting our gut and brain. After eating, try gentle activities like walking or light jogging to help blood flow to your stomach and digestion. This aids in good digestion and regular bowel movements. Breaking up your walk into short sessions can boost blood flow and heart rate. Doing leg and stomach exercises can help your bowels work better. And **remember**, skipping rope workouts during breaks can be surprisingly effective.

As we age, our cells' powerhouses, called mitochondria, may not work as well due to stress, inflammation, and genetics. While it is true, they might not work as efficiently as before, ageing and how mitochondria function are complex processes we are still learning about.

Gut-friendly yoga poses

Try doing easy yoga poses that target your stomach and help you relax, like cat-cow, child's pose, and seated forward bend. These poses can ease tension in your stomach and improve digestion.

Deep breathing exercises

When you practice deep breathing exercises like stomach breathing, you stimulate the vagus nerve. This nerve connects your gut, and the brain controls many bodily functions, including digestion. Deep breathing activates the parasympathetic nervous system, called the 'rest and digest' mode. This triggers a relaxation response in your body, calming your digestive system. This can significantly help with IBS symptoms such as bloating and discomfort.

Tai chi movements

Tai chi involves slow, gentle movements that can relax your stomach and improve digestion. You can practice Tai chi moves like "wave hands like clouds" or "parting wild horse's mane" daily, even in short sessions. It is better to do a little than nothing at all. Mix it up and try different moves for variety. **Tip:** it is not ideal to do the same moves with the same intensity all the time. Instead, try different moves, vary your practice times, and adjust the intensity for better results. Stay fully focused and present during your practice, whether exercise or rituals, for better results.

Pilates for core strength

Building strong core muscles can improve your posture and ease pressure on your digestive system. Pilates exercises like the hundred, pelvic curl, and leg circles are ideal as they won't strain your abdomen too much.

Water-based exercises

Try water-based exercises, like swimming or water aerobics. They give your body gentle resistance and support. The water's buoyancy can ease pressure on your abdomen and give you a low-impact workout option if you have IBS.

Always pay attention to your body's feelings and avoid exercises that worsen your symptoms. If you have other underlying health issues, seek professional guidance from a healthcare professional before starting any new exercises.

What is a healthy weight, BMI and body fat for IBS management

A healthy weight means being at a weight that is right for your body, making you feel good and reducing the chance of health issues. It is different for everyone because it considers factors like how tall and old you are, and your body composition, such as the proportion of muscle, fat, bone, and other tissues. Doctors sometimes use Body Mass Index (BMI) to get an idea of your weight, but it is not always accurate or holistic. Eating well, staying active, and feeling happy and strong are more important than just your weight number.

BMI Range	Category
Less than 18.5	Underweight
18.5 to 24.9	Healthy weight
25.0 to 29.9	Overweight
30.0 or higher	Obese

Self-created table by Jan Nallathamby. Content from The Centers for Disease Control and Prevention 'How to Measure and Interpret Weight Status'

BMI looks at your weight and your height and does not measure fat. It gives a general idea if your weight is right for you. BMI does not distinguish between fat and muscle. For instance, bodybuilders often have a high BMI due to their muscle mass, not body fat. BMI can incorrectly categorise them as obese, even though they are very fit and healthy. While BMI is a quick way to check if you are at a healthy weight, it is most effective to use it with other health checks from your doctor to get a complete picture of your health. **Tip:** a healthcare professional with training should conduct necessary health assessments to check a person's health and understand potential risks.

How using a digital smart scale helps manage IBS through calorie and fat monitoring

A digital body fat smart scale is a helpful tool for managing IBS. It tells you more than just your weight. It shows your body fat percentage and BMR, which is how many calories your body needs at rest each day. A personal helpful recommendation, 'Bluetooth Body Fat Scales, INSMART Smart Digital Bathroom Weight Weighing Scales for Body Composition Analyser with Smart APP, Body Composition Fitbit Scales for Fitness, ' click here, is available on Amazon. Alternatively, check the 'Additional Resources' chapter for the complete link.

These smart scales, like the one suggested above, automatically connect to apps like the 'Insmart Health ' app on your phone. The app tracks your data over time, such as body water, visceral fat, bone mass, BMR, body age, protein, fat level, body type, lean body mass, standard weight, skeletal muscle, and subcutaneous fat, and give you personalised health tips. For someone with IBS, having a record of body changes, dietary habits, and IBS flare-ups can help you spot what triggers your symptoms and what helps reduce them.

This helps you plan your diet better, ensuring you get enough nutrients without overeating. Using an intelligent scale regularly lets you see how your diet and lifestyle affect your body composition, which can inform dietary adjustments. **Key takeaway:** if your body fat percentage goes down and your BMR is improving, your new habits are working. This helps you plan the most suitable diet and make lifestyle choices for optimal gut health.

Bonus tip: instead of worrying only about body fat, focus on living a healthy lifestyle overall.

Knowing your body fat percentage helps you monitor your health. Too much body fat can exacerbate IBS symptoms.

	Body Fat Percentage Range	Recommended Daily Calorie Intake
Men	8-22%	1800-2500 calories
Women	15-20%	1400-2000 calories
Children (2 to 19 years)	10-25%	1000-1400 calories

Self-created table by Jan Nallathamby. Content from The Centers for Disease Control and Prevention

The body fat percentage, daily recommended calorie intake table, smart scale, and SMART app can help you track your overall health. Your body fat and calorie needs vary with age and activity level, and these tools assist you in making necessary adjustments.

Splitting your resting metabolic rate and energy expenditure into smaller meals throughout the day results in smaller portions. This approach is beneficial for IBS and can help reduce postpartum depression. Since breastfeeding women only need 200-600 extra calories, it shows that adults often eat more than necessary.

It is important to watch portion sizes, especially with rising obesity rates. Too much body fat and large portions can make IBS symptoms like inflammation, diarrhoea, constipation, and bloating worse. Using an intelligent body fat digital scale to monitor body fat helps you aim for a healthier BMI and better gut health.

Key point: eat nutritious, varied, balanced foods daily rather than just trying to lose or gain weight. Eating smaller, balanced meals makes it easier for your stomach to handle, which is particularly helpful for managing IBS.

Keep an eye on your waist circumference, which is critical for managing IBS symptoms and gut health. Your health could be in danger if:

	Danger Zone	Greater Risk Zone
Women	>32 inches (80cm)	>35 inches (88cm)
Men	>37 inches (94cm)	> inches (94cm)

Self-created table by Jan Nallathamby. Content from The Centers for Disease Control and Prevention 'Waist Circumference'

Building muscle and reducing unhealthy fat around the waist through exercise, monitored by tracking skeletal muscle and lean body mass in the Insmart health app discussed earlier, is essential for managing IBS. It can promote gut health and enhance digestion. **Bonus tip:** eating based on what science says, instead of just following cultural or emotional cues, can also help. It means focusing on balanced meals that are good for your gut.

After exercising, consume natural sources of protein rather than protein shakes, sports bars, sports drinks, gels and supplement powders, as they can contain lactose, fructose, and unsuitable sweeteners and also can be harsh on the sensitive gut, potentially affecting the microbiome health. Whey protein isolate has very little lactose, so it may suit most individuals, even those sensitive to lactose. It is ideal to eat your protein rather than drink it. Natural protein sources can aid in muscle recovery and improve IBS symptoms. Exercise makes you feel good by releasing endorphins, sometimes called 'happy hormones.' These chemicals can lift your mood and lower stress, which can help with managing IBS symptoms.

Trying mindfulness during meals, like paying close attention to how your body reacts to different foods, can also help manage IBS symptoms better.

Understanding your calorie and protein needs

Seeking guidance from a healthcare professional is invaluable when managing IBS symptoms, providing a sense of security and support. For instance, a TDEE (Total Daily Energy Expenditure) calorie calculator can assist in determining your daily calorie requirements. Target about 0.8 grams of protein per kilogram of body weight daily, sourced from both vegetarian and non-vegetarian foods. After a workout, adults should consume 15-20 grams of protein to aid muscle recovery. Children may require less protein, so it is wise to follow this guideline unless advised otherwise by a healthcare professional.

CHAPTER RECAP:

This chapter emphasises the pivotal role of exercise, a balanced diet, and monitoring calorie intake and body fat percentage in managing IBS symptoms. It reminds us that we have the power to influence our health. A healthy weight and BMI are crucial, and using a digital smart scale can track progress and offer personalised health tips for those managing IBS symptoms.

Monitoring portion sizes and focusing on nutritious, balanced meals based on science, not emotions or cultural cues, are essential for managing IBS symptoms. This guidance can provide reassurance and a sense of being on the right track. Paying attention to protein intake and avoiding protein supplements can support sensitive gut health and muscle recovery.

As we age, our bodies become less efficient at producing energy, reducing physical strength and gut health. To counteract this, it is important to include weight training, eat a varied diet, and keep track of exercise routines. These habits can help maintain optimal energy levels, stay strong, and improve overall health and quality of life as we age.

Exercise, particularly gentle activities and yoga, can be beneficial for digestion and relieving stomach tension. Deep breathing exercises have the potential to stimulate the Vagus nerve, which in turn calms the digestive system. Consistent practice of Tai chi, pilates, and water-based exercises, coupled with a positive mindset, can also contribute to improved gut health.

Focus on a healthy waist circumference rather than just trying to lose or gain weight. Smaller, balanced meal portions are more accessible to the digestive system and can help manage IBS. Exercise, proper nutrition, and mindful eating are not just strategies; they are powerful tools that can significantly improve gut health and well-being.

Balancing Personal Well-Being With Professional Excellence

"Earth provides enough to satisfy every man's needs, but not every man's greed." — *Mahatma Gandhi*

In this chapter, you will learn how to care for yourself while doing great at your job. It talks about having a positive mindset and discipline, managing your time and energy well, reducing stress at work, communicating effectively, setting boundaries at work and home, and quick tips for managing IBS flare-ups at home.

21. Abundance Mindset and Discipline

"All great ideas are dangerous." — Oscar Wilde

It is essential to start your day with a purpose and end it with gratitude. You might spend most of your time at work, so ensuring your career is what makes you content is critical for overall health. Health drives your work and brings the money you need, so your career and IBS management are linked. Much of this depends on having an abundance mindset, which means thinking positively and believing in endless possibilities, along with discipline.

Having an abundance mindset means looking at life positively in your thoughts, words and actions. It can help with IBS because it makes you focus on what is good in your life, which reduces stress. Discipline is essential as well. It enables you to stick to healthy habits that ease IBS symptoms to create an impactful life. It helps you stay on track at work, even when dealing with IBS challenges. By staying positive and disciplined, you can manage IBS better and excel in your career.

Assessing your career fit and well-being

Is your career the right choice for you in the long term? Take a 10-minute free personality test to see if your job boosts your energy and brings in a healthy stress level. That is key for those with IBS for handling microbiome dysbiosis. You can find the test at psality.com/test-en/, accessed by clicking here. This test can help you figure out if your job is right for you and if it makes you happy. To plan for a fulfilling future, practice having an abundance mindset towards yourself and others daily, even when facing various inevitable life challenges. You grow multi-fold if those around you grow as much as you do. Allocate dedicated time, free from distractions, to focus on planning your future, considering your career goals and managing your IBS health.

Managing anxiety and career direction

Try not to dwell too much on the pains of IBS, as it can affect your ability to think clearly. Stay positive and believe that focusing on the good things in life can lead to more positivity and better IBS symptom management. The dynamic, fast-paced world we live in today calls for some inner focus and trusting the process. It is like how we trust the pilot or the driver we never knew to safely get us to our destination. When you are worried about where your career is headed, which is a healthy thought at any stage, take a moment to step back, stay detached and be gentle with yourself. Try to remain calm and show yourself some kindness, as anxiety can lead to stress. **Remember**, what you studied for and working on may not always lead directly to your career or success. Life's path is not always straightforward, but believing in yourself will pay off. Your path may twist and turn, but you will reach your goals eventually. Your choices shape your destiny, so live with purpose, yet lightly, and always follow your moral compass.

Aligning career with well-being

We aim to understand whether our current career fits well with our IBS situation and whether it is necessary to consider changing careers to find optimal peace and fulfilment. Believe in the possibility and create your own path forward because only you have the power to make it happen.

Sometimes, the answers come to you when you least expect it, like during a game of golf or a post-lunch walk. Stay strong by lifting weights, keep your heart healthy with cardio, and stretch your muscles for flexibility. Read to learn, write to reflect, and be creative. Be grateful, spend time in nature, and meditate for peace. Every day, see if you can spare 5 minutes for each activity, even during your busiest times.

Cultivating a positive mindset and self-awareness

Be mindful of maintaining positive and abundant thoughts, as they can significantly impact your subconscious mind and ultimately affect your health, work, and overall life.

Research Ikigai, a Japanese concept, and mark what makes you happy with a smiley face and what you can get paid for with a currency sign. Choose the option that has both signs and matches your beliefs and values, as it might be your most suitable choice for your career. Focus on fulfilling your soul, not just meeting society's expectations.

Focusing on blessings and priorities

Do not worry. Be patient and focus on your current blessings and priorities in life. Instead of letting fears overwhelm you, stay calm and keep your blessings and priorities, such as personal projects, family, friends, and inner happiness, at the forefront of your mind.

Embracing life's illusion and finding real peace

Ultimately, life is like an illusion that fades away when your soul leaves your body. People will only remember how you made them feel in the end. This means staying humble and true to yourself is the key to finding real peace, which leads to health and happiness in every aspect of your life. Remember, it is not just the facts but the stories we tell ourselves that can lead to procrastination and negativity in our minds. We are our most prominent critics. Surround yourself with positive individuals and trust a higher power to guide you. Seek help from those you prefer who can be your critical friend and build a support team that wants to see you succeed. Create a promising future for yourself and appreciate the journey, not just the end goal, by embracing the concept of magical fallacy.

Balancing personal well-being with professional excellence

This stresses how essential it is to feel happy in your job regularly since you spend most of your life working, with sleep being the only activity that possibly surpasses it. Assess where you are currently and start building momentum with small steps, as they can lead to more significant achievements through a domino effect. As we discussed, meal planning and diet are also about variety, portion control, and consistency. The same applies to an abundant mindset with discipline for balancing personal well-being with professional excellence.

Professional excellence is important because it leads to high-quality work and helps achieve personal and company goals. Working with joyful colleagues who love their jobs and, for some, working with the top in their field also helps. It builds trust and respect with co-workers and clients, opening doors for better opportunities and career growth. Aiming for excellence gives a sense of achievement and happiness, which adds to overall success and well-being. This includes stress management for those with IBS, as unhealthy stress can trigger IBS symptoms.

Setting career goals for IBS health management

If you are up for a challenge, think big and envision where you want to be in the next 10 years. Then, work backwards to 5 and 3 years, breaking it down into yearly, quarterly, monthly, weekly, and daily goals. This method keeps you driven and motivated, leading to tremendous success in the long run with your health and your career.

Create a business or look for jobs that let you choose your hours. This way, you can manage IBS symptoms and stress better. Find a career with less stress. High-stress jobs can worsen IBS symptoms, so it is wise to work in peaceful environments like your home, around nature or a café, or wherever that suits your IBS health needs. Choose colleagues who prioritise health and well-being by discussing them transparently. You might as well work with the right colleagues who want to build you as much as build mutual purpose and profit margins. They might offer benefits like nutrition advice and mental health support, which can help with IBS and overall health.

Taking action and overcoming setbacks

Be disciplined and stick to a plan of discovering if your career is right for you using Ikigai and the personality test discussed above. If long-term planning is not for you, you can still make small changes to switch careers or move at any age or stage. It is all about having a positive mindset and taking calculated risks based on what brings you joy and purpose, which results from finding your Ikigai. Even if it is just spending fifteen minutes each day, think of the end result, such as more peace and better IBS health, and work backwards to figure out your Ikigai.

Just take action today, and you will get better along the way. **Key takeaway:** take action today in small chunks, and take your time. Once you start, it will become easier and begin to have a domino effect in all aspects of life, such as IBS food trackers and morning and night routines. It is expected to slip up a few days or weeks, just get back on track. Having accountability partners can help make the journey enjoyable so it feels effortless. Choose what works effectively for you personally. There is no one-size-fits-all approach; everyone might take different paths to reach their goals. The key is to have a positive mindset towards yourself and support others on their journey to positivity. Celebrate the clarity you find in discovering the right career for you. **Personal tip:** I have discovered that taking on new challenges is essential because growth and comfort cannot coexist. **Remember,** there is always time to change, regardless of age. Some individuals prefer to stay where they are, and that is okay. It is important to respect personal choices and support them in that, too.

CHAPTER RECAP:

Starting your day with a purpose and ending it with gratitude is essential, especially since we spend a lot of time working. Your job and managing IBS are connected. Having a positive mindset and being disciplined are critical to this.

Assessing your job and well-being is essential. A short free test at psality.com/test-en/ can help you see if your job makes you happy and elevates your energy. A positive attitude and setting career goals considering your IBS requirements can lead to a balanced life.

Being passionate and excellent at your job matters for your happiness and managing stress, especially if you have IBS. Working with positive individuals and focusing on health at work can help immensely.

Setting career goals that suit your IBS needs, like choosing flexible hours or low-stress jobs, can help manage symptoms. Overcoming challenges and working towards your purpose can lead to a fulfilling life.

Consistently taking small actions can trigger positive results, especially when you prioritise yourself and inspire others to do the same. This approach leads to a clearer perspective, improving your mindset, discipline, sense of purpose, personal well-being, and professional success.

Remember the magical fallacy, as there is always time to make a single correct decision that can change it all for your health, and celebrating your progress along the way is essential.

Ultimately, maintaining a positive outlook, being disciplined with a system that suits your life, and gradually working towards your goals around all areas of your life where you lead by example can have a significant impact on your life and those around you, creating a ripple effect of positive changes, even when dealing with IBS.

22. Time and Energy Management

"Great minds have purpose, others have wishes." — Washington Irving

Life is all about time and energy management through discipline. Managing your time and energy well can significantly help with IBS when balancing personal well-being with professional excellence. When you organise your tasks and take breaks, it can lower your stress. Less stress means fewer IBS symptoms. When you plan your day, you can make time for healthy habits like eating well and relaxing, which are crucial for managing IBS. By managing your time wisely, you are getting more done and taking better care of yourself and your gut health. Good time management allows you to get more done and still have time to recharge over the weekend with family and friends. **Key takeaway:** how you spend your weekends shapes your week. If you feel you are losing balance, quickly regain it before it affects your health and worsens your IBS symptoms. Let's delve deeper into how we can accomplish this.

Time vs energy management

Time is limited and not within our control, but our energy is renewable and manageable. Managing time involves eliminating distractions while managing energy means being mindful of when distractions affect us. Prioritise tasks that yield the most significant impact and energise us.

An energy audit helps us understand how to manage our daily energy better, leading to improved health and productivity. To perform an energy audit, track your daily activities, meals, sleep, and energy levels. Identify patterns to adjust your routine for more energy-boosting and less energy-draining activities. Monitor your energy levels and make adjustments to maintain a balanced lifestyle. For example, having a green smoothie, a quick 20-minute walk followed by a jog post lunch or a mid-day 20-minute power nap can boost productivity. Stay focused on the present moment to make time for self-care activities throughout the day, ensuring you feel valued and cared for.

The locus of control, developed by Julian B. Rotter in 1954, refers to whether we believe our outcomes are influenced by internal actions or external factors like luck. Focusing on what we can control, such as our actions and decisions, is crucial for energy management. Recognising our four energy buckets - mental, physical, emotional, and spiritual—helps us prioritise tasks and understand that progress takes time. This understanding of control over our energy can empower us to make positive changes in our lives.

The Habit Scorecard, a tool developed by James Clear, is a powerful way to track daily habits. It helps identify positive, negative, or neutral behaviours, allowing you to focus on reducing negative and enhancing positive habits. This leads to better decision-making and increased productivity. Energy vampires, whether individuals, locations, or objects, can drain your energy. It is wise to avoid them and instead focus on positive influences that uplift your spirits. With practice, this becomes effortless. **Personal tip:** start tackling the most critical task within an hour of waking up, as that's when most individuals tend to be most productive.

For more insights on building habits, consider reading "Atomic Habits" by James Clear, available on Amazon click here. Check the 'Additional Resources' chapter for the complete link. The book explores how consistent application of the Habit Loop and principles of behaviour change can lead to lasting improvements over time. By learning about the Habit Loop, which is a cue, craving, response, reward, and using behaviour change principles such as making habits clear, appealing, easy, and satisfying, Clear gives practical ways for individuals to change their habits and improve their daily routines. For example, sticking to regular meals, eating foods high in fibre, drinking enough water, and handling stress well are all based on forming good habits that ease symptoms and make life better for those with IBS. To stop bad habits, make them hard to notice, unappealing, challenging, and not rewarding. Clear also highlights the significance of identity, advising that aiming to become the person you want to be can bring about long-term change. The book offers practical guidance and real-world examples to help readers use these ideas in their own lives.

Connecting with future self

Visualise your future self by imagining a better version of who you want to be. It helps you concentrate on tasks that move you closer to your long-term goals. Start your day positively and imagine how you want to make a difference in the world. Consistently taking action can lead to significant changes in your life and society, giving you a sense of accomplishment and motivation.

Imagine a personal wellness plan where each daily task contributes towards your long-term goals. This progress builds over time, much like compound interest, shaping the future you have envisioned for yourself.

Every individual has the power to make a positive impact, not only in their own life but also in the world around them. This happens when they find joy in their career, maintain a positive mindset, utilise their time effectively, and channel their energy wisely towards meaningful pursuits.

You can positively impact the world by prioritising your IBS health, reducing stress, and remaining committed to your career and personal objectives.

Creating momentum with small, focused steps and intentional play

Start with your goals for the day, set realistic expectations to avoid stress, and be kind to yourself. You are already enough. Limit it to three goals that would help your long-term growth in all areas of your life, and then plan the steps to get there. Allocate 20 minutes to one hour for each goal. Let others know about your goals so they can support you mentally, emotionally, and spiritually. This could be a trusted sisterhood, brotherhood, or a supportive friend who pushes you to be your best and serves as your constructive critic. This support can come in different ways: giving you space at work and home or offering encouragement and positivity.

Divide your goals into smaller tasks and integrate them into your daily schedule. This way, you can see how to reach your objectives step by step. **Tip:** think about the bigger purpose behind combining work with intentional play daily, like engaging in activities opposite your career to sharpen various parts of your brain. For instance, if you are in finance, consider dedicating 15 minutes each day to hobbies like painting, writing or playing the guitar. While it might seem short, even this time can make a difference compared to not doing it at all. These activities should be integrated with your daily career and health goals to nurture creativity, self-expression, memory, and patience, ultimately promoting overall well-being and potentially reducing IBS symptoms. These muscles need regular workouts to stay strong as you age.

Build stronger relationships with more time for family and friends that strengthen personal bonds and elevate your health. This helps you feel less stressed and more energised when you return to work. Occasionally, consider volunteering at places like nature reserves or animal shelters or joining spiritual causes to lead a more fulfilling life. Balance your career, health and personal goals evenly throughout the week and be mindful of how you use your time. Time is a valuable resource that often goes unnoticed. Just like managing your energy, prioritise your most important tasks when your energy levels are high and save the less important ones for later in the day when your energy dips if that is the case for you.

Small steps lead to significant achievements through a domino effect. Include a mix of work and personal activities with short breaks in your daily schedule to prevent burnout and keep it light and enjoyable. This can help increase energy without straining your body. Treat yourself when you reach your goals. Use your phone's note-taking feature to jot down tasks and enjoy the satisfaction of checking them off as you complete them.

Ideal flexibility discipline

Striking a balance between flexible and structured routines is critical to managing IBS when achieving long-term success in your career. Flexibility allows you to adapt to the unpredictable nature of IBS flare-ups and life's complexities, focusing on high-value priorities across health, career, and personal goals daily. Incorporate activities like deep work sessions or regular exercise into your schedule to improve productivity. Discipline ensures you stick to healthy habits discussed in earlier sections that reduce IBS discomfort, allowing you to effectively manage your workload when your energy swings throughout the day. Prioritise self-care activities such as gut-directed hypnotherapy for IBS management, a warm bubble bath to relax muscles or journaling to focus on what matters so you can pass on the rest. This well-rounded approach helps with your overall well-being, balancing the demands of your career and managing IBS symptoms.

Some experts recommend daily writing, while others suggest avoiding skipping tasks for two days in a row. My routine includes writing before checking work emails, doing short exercises for flexibility and strength, and self-care sessions while enjoying nature. Try 20 minutes of intense exercise thrice weekly or two short walks in nature when you are busy.

Managing energy is essential for those with IBS. Maintain hydration and consume balanced small meals for steady energy levels, which are essential for a balanced career. It is expected that you will work too hard and realise your body cannot keep up with the pace of your mind or vice versa. You want to aim for harmony between your time, energy, mind, and body for optimal health and performance in your career.

If you manage your energy levels and time wisely, you can ease IBS symptoms, which helps your health and work performance. Set time in the day to do nothing for at least 20 minutes for self-reflection.

Trust but verify mentality

It means you trust things to be reliable, but you also take steps to check and make sure they are accurate and trustworthy. For instance, using tools like the 'Opal: Screen Time for Focus' app helps you avoid distractions from social media, which can improve your ability to concentrate and get tasks done effectively. It is about using technology to help you stay focused on important tasks and not waste time on things that can distract you.

Set a timer on your phone to restrict social media scrolling to half an hour or less once or twice daily. Avoid checking multiple times throughout the day and refrain from spending too much time on social media first thing in the morning or late at night. It is ideal to browse social media when you are feeling low on energy, although this varies for each person. As mentioned, scrolling before bed can disrupt your sleep and affect your IBS health, even with a healthy diet. It is about finding the right balance and consistently making intelligent choices. Social media and movies can be addictive, so it is wise to use your time wisely. Avoid excessive scrolling through others' content outside your set daily time limit. Instead, focus on your goals to advance your career and enhance your personal life.

CHAPTER RECAP:

This chapter discusses how managing time and energy can help with IBS symptoms and improve overall well-being. It suggests organising tasks, taking breaks, and focusing on healthy habits to reduce stress and improve gut health. Good career time management, by following your peak energy levels, also allows for quality time with loved ones on weekends, which sets a positive tone for the week ahead.

Maintaining a "trust but verify" mindset helps stay focused, with tools like the 'Opal: Screen Time for Focus' app being helpful. Setting limits on social media use and prioritising personal goals over passive scrolling can boost productivity and self-improvement. Engaging in hobbies unrelated to work promotes creativity and well-being, which can reduce IBS symptoms.

Balancing flexibility and discipline is essential for managing IBS and succeeding in one's career. Flexibility helps adapt to life's challenges, while discipline ensures sticking to healthy habits. Prioritising self-care activities like gut-directed hypnotherapy and maintaining a balance between work and good health contributes to overall well-being that further fuels other areas of life, like your career.

Visualising one's future self and setting long-term goals can foster personal development and positively influence society. Every individual has the power to make a difference by finding joy in their career, staying positive, and managing their time and energy effectively. Strive to keep alert, updated, and active in life's challenges. Individuals can significantly impact the world by focusing on health, reducing stress, and staying committed to goals.

The chapter also emphasises the significance of consistency in actions for significant change, finding a productivity "sweet spot" that balances discipline and flexibility, and prioritising high-value tasks while maintaining a positive outlook. Creating momentum through small steps and establishing effective life systems further supports the journey towards career success for managing your well-being with IBS. Consistency is vital, so keep at it through life's ups and downs.

23. Stress Reduction Work Techniques

"The secret of success is to do the common thing uncommonly well." — John D. Rockefeller Jr.

Stress often worsens IBS symptoms, so managing stress at work is vital for feeling better.

High levels of stress can lead you to neglect dietary habits or coping strategies that usually help manage IBS, worsening the symptoms. Long-term stress can compromise the immune system, increasing vulnerability to infections and diseases. It can also make the gut more sensitive, resulting in more frequent or severe IBS symptoms like cramps and diarrhoea. Stress affects both our minds and bodies, potentially resulting in serious health issues like heart disease, a weakened immune system, digestive problems, and chronic pain.

Various factors influence how stress affects health, including the type, number, and duration of the stressors, as well as individual biological factors such as genetics and overall health, psychological resources, and learned coping mechanisms. Together, these factors determine the impact of stress on disease and well-being.

Knowing what level of stress is too much for you can help, and this can vary with each person based on health, age, life situations and other factors. Therefore, keeping stress in check for your gut health and career performance is essential. Surround yourself with supportive co-workers who create a largely happy and positive atmosphere. When you are in job interviews or working together, clearly talk about your career ambitions and what matters to you regarding stress, IBS and your work. Be honest and transparent, as it will save you more stress in the long term. This helps everyone understand each other better and brings mutual benefits, drawing from insights from your personality and the Ikigai tests we discussed earlier. The more transparent you are with your colleagues, the better. The right work colleagues will appreciate your honesty and align with your IBS situation to support you through your career success.

Communicate with colleagues

If you experience an IBS flare-up, let your colleagues know. Hence, they understand any changes in your energy levels or appearance due to fatigue. **Remember**, focusing on the journey of your career, including its challenges and successes, brings happiness both in your professional life and in managing IBS symptoms. This highlights the importance of acknowledging and managing work-related stress and sharing your experiences so others can better support you.

Relaxation techniques

Using a mindfulness journal, body scanning and meditation, and taking 20-minute power naps, especially during challenging IBS flare-ups at work, can reduce stress and improve overall well-being. This not only improves mood, cognitive function, and work productivity but also provides much-needed relief from the symptoms of IBS. A well-rested mind operates more efficiently, producing sharper thinking and reduced errors. Studies show that these techniques can cut stress when practised consistently and with intention, which is impressive and can help with IBS symptoms to manage work-related stress.

Watching something funny or reading jokes, cartoons, or comics can make you feel better when stressed. It is like a natural mood lifter because it releases chemicals in your body that make you happy. This can be particularly beneficial when managing the difficulties of IBS in the workplace. Taking a break to laugh can give you a mental reset and help you feel more positive, making coping with stress easier. Taking time to enjoy a good laugh can be a simple way to feel better and manage stress, even when you are dealing with IBS at work.

Making these relaxation methods a part of their daily routine can make a big difference in how they feel and improve work productivity.

Taking breaks

Take quick breaks to clear your mind by stepping away from your desk, practice deep breathing with mindfulness or take a short walk for a change in scenery. Try shifting your focus to what you want, not what you do not wish to. This can help you refocus on work tasks and release tension by concentrating on your breath. During work breaks, avoid addictions such as coffee, vaping or smoking. Instead, choose caffeine-free, non-carbonated drinks like a ready-made green smoothie or a homemade millet or nut drink. You can also listen to podcasts with colleagues, discussing intellectual topics and ideas. Avoiding negative talks helps with your IBS stress management.

To relax your muscles at work, tense and then release each muscle group while seated. This aids in progressive muscle relaxation, which can reduce symptoms like stomach cramps, brain fog, or anxiety associated with IBS. **Personal tip:** lower your head towards your knees and gently massage your scalp for a minute to release stress.

Make sure to plan these breaks deliberately in your work calendar. Move around frequently, as movement helps your gut stay active and healthy. Visualise yourself in a serene setting or work next to your garden by focusing on calming images or nature during your breaks.

Using collaboration tools

Collaboration work tools like Slack, Trello, Microsoft Teams, Asana, and Google Workspace can help reduce stress at work by encouraging communication, task management, and project collaboration among team members. Work with your co-workers to split up tasks and support each other when required. This makes the workload lighter and creates a feeling of teamwork and help among everyone. Break tasks into smaller steps, communicate openly with colleagues about workload, and make mutual accommodations where required. This largely depends on how severe your IBS symptoms are, and sometimes flare-ups can occur unexpectedly.

Time management and organisation

Use time management techniques like the Pomodoro technique and keep your workspace organised. Utilising the Pomodoro technique by working for 25 minutes, followed by a short break, and keeping your workspace tidy can help you manage your energy better and reduce stress. When your workspace is neat, it is easier to think clearly, feel less overwhelmed, focus better, and feel in control, which can be especially helpful when dealing with IBS symptoms. By using this technique and keeping things organised, you can work more efficiently and feel less stressed, making it easier to manage your IBS.

Managing over thinking

It is expected to have troubling thoughts and understand that nothing will ever be flawless. Focus on doing your best rather than chasing perfection. Instead of waiting for the perfect moment, take action and get things done. Avoid putting things off, and keep your long-term goals in mind. Trying to be perfect can add stress, which is particularly challenging for individuals dealing with IBS.

Instead of focusing on problems, concentrate on finding solutions. Take each day at a time. Think about the long-term goals and what you can achieve today by being present in the moment. Life can be very uncertain. This proactive method can help reduce anxiety and prevent overthinking, making it easier to manage IBS symptoms. Overthinking about work often leads to increased stress and can worsen IBS symptoms.

Recognise the signs of overthinking, including constant worrying, replaying past events, or imagining worst-case scenarios. If you find yourself stuck in a loop of thoughts, you might be overthinking. Physical symptoms like headaches, muscle tension, and digestive issues can also indicate overthinking. Indecision can add to your stress, making it hard to make decisions because you second-guess yourself constantly. Sleep disruptions, like trouble sleeping or feeling restless at night, can also be a sign of overthinking, and lack of sleep can make IBS symptoms worse. This can increase stress and affect gut health. When you are not hindered by excessive thoughts, you can focus better on your work and daily tasks, leading to higher productivity and less stress. By managing overthinking, you can help maintain better physical health.

Bonus tip: to manage to overthink, set time limits for thinking about a problem. Once the time is up, move on to action or let it go. Focus on aspects of your work and life that you can influence. Let go of things beyond your control. On tough days, remind yourself with positive thoughts like "I get to do this" instead of "I have to do this." This quickly shifts your mindset and makes you feel lighter and less stressed. If using "I" does not feel impactful when talking to yourself, try using your name or a third-person perspective. For instance, instead of saying, *"I feel miserable, but I've faced worse before, so I can handle this,"* try saying, *"I understand you're feeling miserable right now, but you've shown resilience in the past. You have the strength to tackle this new challenge as well."*

Seek support by talking to a colleague, friend, or therapist about your worries. Sometimes, sharing your thoughts can provide new perspectives and reduce the load on your mind. Journaling helps you process your thoughts and feelings, provides clarity, and helps you let go of persistent worries.

Accepting imperfection, focusing on solutions, and managing overthinking can significantly reduce stress and improve your IBS symptoms. This leads to a healthier, more productive work life.

Maintaining work-life balance through smart work

Make sure you have clear limits between work time and personal time so that stress from work does not affect your personal life. Cut out or reduce checking work emails or taking calls when off work. Mention your working hours on your work e-signature for attention and stick to it. Intentionally choose to work with those who can accommodate your IBS health requirements. Follow your personal goals for fulfilment in other areas of life, along with daily self-care. **Remember** that even just 15 minutes can significantly affect different areas of your life, benefiting your work. Celebrate the little wins as you go and enjoy the journey.

Keeping stress-relief tools nearby

Keep stress-relief tools near your work desk, like stress balls or essential oils, to help during tense moments. Be mindful of how your body responds to various foods and drinks, especially when experiencing unhealthy work stress. You can identify which foods trigger your IBS by tracking your diet in a food diary that can help manage symptoms, as discussed earlier, along with the morning routine of journaling your thoughts. This way, you can make smarter choices to better manage your diet, workload, and stress symptoms at work.

To ease work-related anxiety , use oils like lavender, which are known for their calming effects and for reducing stress. Select the right scent and place it carefully for effective aromatherapy at work. Use electric diffusers or gently spray oil mixes on soft fabrics. Position diffusers centrally, about two feet above the floor, and at least three feet away from your colleagues. Use scents that suit different areas, such as calming ones for relaxation and energising scents for workspaces.

Proactive measures for addressing work-related stress with IBS

To kick-start your day positively, stick to the morning routines we discussed in the previous chapter, 'Morning and Night Routine for Gut Health and Well-being.' Make it a habit to follow these routines regularly, and concentrate on things you can influence and be grateful for.

Incorporate the below techniques into your daily routine or use them whenever you feel stressed or anxious at work. Practice mindfulness, swimming, crossword puzzles to divert your mind from work-related stress, meditation in the morning or before bed, and use aromatherapy or positive visualisation during stressful work moments. Sometimes, stress can make you and your gut more sensitive to smells when you have IBS. Choose what suits your needs, such as skipping aromatherapy and going for a walk. **Key takeaway:** avoid allowing work-related stress to persist for multiple days. Instead, talk about your thoughts to get more clarity, which helps reduce overthinking. Practice open communication and establish clear boundaries at work, which we will discuss further in the next chapter to support individuals with IBS. Ask for help when required, and you will appreciate the support.

Further resources to help manage work stress

When you are feeling overwhelmed at work or need assistance with your work relationships:
- If it suits your career, consider working fully remotely or in a hybrid setup to reduce pressure from work or personal relationships.
- Reach out to a mentor, join work-related groups or forums led by a health coach, or consider hiring a consultant for support.
- Explore online courses, self-help books, coaching or counselling services to manage stress effectively.

- Contact your HR department or employee assistance program for tailored guidance on managing work-related stress and IBS symptoms if employed. These resources support your well-being and improve your overall stress management.

For stress management, consider reading the book "The Body Keeps the Score: Mind, Brain, and Body in the Transformation of Trauma.", available on Amazon click here

If childhood stress affects your IBS, check out the book "The Deepest Well: Healing the Long-Term Effects of Childhood Adversity." It is also available on Amazon. Click here

CHAPTER RECAP:

Managing stress at work is very important for those with IBS because stress can make symptoms worse, such as gut sensitivity, irregular bowel movements, worsened anxiety and depression, and also weaken the immune system.

To manage the above, it is imperative to set the tone for the day by following the morning routines we discussed in the chapter 'Morning and Night Routine for Gut Health and Well-being'. Tell your colleagues about your IBS condition so they can support you by covering for you or assisting with deadlines during unexpected flare-ups. Share your career goals and values with your team to ensure mutual understanding and support. Aim for balance rather than perfection at work, as striving for flawlessness can cause anxiety and stress, which may negatively affect your gut health.

Relaxation techniques like mindfulness, meditation, and watching comedy shows can help reduce stress and improve your overall feelings. During IBS flare-ups, taking power naps can also help. Regular work breaks are essential; schedule them with reminders on your phone or work calendar. Use them for deep breathing, short walks, and avoiding coffee or smoking. Instead, choose caffeine-free drinks like green tea, matcha, homemade millet and nut beverages or green smoothies. Moving around often helps keep your gut healthy, especially if you have a desk job.

Discover the importance of letting things go and find inspiration in books that set positive goals. Take a deep breath and reflect on your purpose, known as Ikigai, discussed earlier. Your ambitions to stay motivated and focused.

Keep stress-relief tools like stress balls or essential oils handy for tense moments. Use calming natural scents like lavender for relaxation areas and energising scents for workspaces. Managing not to overthink is also vital. Concentrate on solutions instead of dwelling on problems. Set time limits for thinking about issues and then move on to action. Using your name instead of "I" when talking to yourself can help you better support yourself.

Use collaboration and communication tools like Slack, Trello, and Asana to improve teamwork and reduce stress. Be mindful of your diet; keep a food diary to track what triggers your IBS symptoms; avoid comfort eating by reminding yourself of the consequences and make better food choices. To prevent comfort eating, plan your work snacks ahead with foods that are gentle on your IBS, using the advice from the 'Meal Planning for IBS: Tips and Tricks' chapter. Since IBS flare-ups can occur unexpectedly, preparing healthy snacks can help you manage symptoms when work stress arises. Ensure you have regular small portions of snacks and meals, like high-fibre pre-packed home-sprouted salads and superfoods. These also help individuals with IBS who experience constipation by promoting regular bowel movements.

Consider working remotely or in a hybrid setup if it suits your career. Seek support from mentors, health coaches, or HR departments for help with managing work-related stress and IBS. Additional resources like the books "The Body Keeps the Score" and "The Deepest Well" can offer more insights into handling stress and its impact on health. Focus on your journey, celebrate small wins, and enjoy the process to improve your outlook and manage stress better.

By adding these strategies to your daily routine, you can better manage stress at work, improve your IBS symptoms, and have a healthier, more productive work life.

24. Communication Skills with Setting Boundaries at Work and Home

"Either define the moment or the moment will define you." — Walt Whitman

Managing IBS with effective communication and boundary setting is critical for balancing personal well-being with professional excellence. This section covers how these skills can smooth the journey amidst the challenges of IBS.

IBS has a significant effect on everyday life and productivity. A survey from April to June 2022 collected data from 1,800 people aged 18-25. Most of the participants were females (53%) from Saudi Arabia. On average, individuals with IBS lose about two days of productivity each month due to their symptoms. Those who work more than nine hours a day, especially in sedentary jobs, are more likely to develop IBS. Over half of the people surveyed found their symptoms very bothersome.

Different types of IBS have other impacts. Those with IBS-C often avoid sex, find it difficult to concentrate and feel self-conscious. Meanwhile, individuals with IBS-D tend to avoid places without toilets, have trouble planning, stay home more often, and are hesitant to travel.

In summary, IBS causes many issues, affecting quality of life and work. Moreover, individuals with IBS who experience high levels of anxiety and depression may have suicidal thoughts due to their symptoms, highlighting the severity of the condition. Raising awareness about your IBS at school, home, work, and in social circles is crucial. Communicating openly and setting clear boundaries can help others understand your condition and support your well-being.

Consequences of not setting clear boundaries when managing IBS

When you have IBS, not setting clear boundaries can cause extra stress and discomfort. It might lead to over-committing yourself or feeling pressured, making it harder to manage symptoms. Clear boundaries are essential because they help you manage your time and energy better, which is crucial when dealing with a sensitive condition like IBS.

For those with IBS, it is crucial to communicate clearly and set firm boundaries. This helps others understand your needs and protects your mental, emotional, and physical well-being. Together, they form a roadmap for navigating the complexities of IBS.

From helping yourself to communicating

To effectively manage IBS, start by speaking up early about recurring abdominal pain and bowel issues rather than dealing with them alone. Describe your symptoms thoroughly, including how they affect your daily life and what treatments you have tried. Keep your doctor informed if symptoms persist despite treatment to explore other options for relief.

Talking openly about your IBS with others is crucial for gaining their understanding and support. Identify triggers and establish clear boundaries to manage your condition effectively. **Tip:** in new relationships or situations, use "I" statements to express your needs clearly and honestly, promoting empathy and understanding. Actively listen to others to strengthen relationships and create a supportive environment.

Stay in touch regularly with your support network, such as family or close colleagues, to keep them informed and adjust your routine as needed. Aim for regular conversations to maintain open communication and promptly address any concerns.

Setting boundaries to help manage IBS better

Individuals with IBS tend to be more sensitive to their bowel movements, which can make them feel pain more quickly. This sensitivity can affect their ability to handle stress at work because the pain and unpredictability of symptoms might make it hard to focus or perform tasks. Clear communication of boundaries is essential in these situations to help colleagues understand and offer support without causing further discomfort.

Having supportive relationships is crucial for managing IBS. People with strong support networks often find their symptoms relieved and work better when they have chronic health conditions. Having friends, family, or a community to lean on can make a big difference in how they cope with their illness. This support can provide emotional comfort and practical help, improving their overall well-being. It highlights the value of having understanding and caring people around you when dealing with this condition.

It is crucial to clearly define your limits and priorities at work and home, ensuring they support your health goals to avoid burnout. Start by identifying what matters most to you in both your work and personal life. Ask yourself questions like 'What qualities do I appreciate in other relationships?', 'Which material items are most important to me and why?' and 'What gives me a sense of fulfillment?' Then, prioritise how you use your time and energy according to these priorities. For instance, you might prioritise positivity, the option to work remotely or smartly rather than just hard wherever possible and communicate these boundaries clearly but politely, particularly concerning remote work, which can be beneficial if you encounter immunity issues that may arise for some with IBS. **Personal tip:** positive relationships are vital. Handle stressful or unsupportive remarks calmly but firmly when the timing is appropriate. Clearly explain how their words affect you and suggest ways they can offer more helpful support in the future. Journaling and practising better communication at work and home can help articulate your needs regarding IBS management and improve physical and emotional support. Asking for assistance rather than facing challenges silently is vital to managing stress and maintaining healthy boundaries in daily life.

Confident boundaries help maintain a balanced life, enabling effective prioritisation and lowering stress. Establishing boundaries early, especially in demanding situations like work pressure or social commitments, supports effective prioritisation and overall well-being, including gut health and managing IBS symptoms.

Setting boundaries ensures time for crucial self-care activities such as rest, exercise, and healthy eating. Adequate sleep and consistent physical activity are vital for gut health, facilitated by clear boundaries. This approach protects mental well-being and minimises stress. Assertively communicating these boundaries includes declining commitments when necessary, such as work demands or social pressures, promoting overall balance and IBS health management.

CHAPTER RECAP:

Effective management of IBS involves mastering communication skills and establishing clear boundaries, which are vital for balancing personal well-being with professional success. This chapter discussed how these skills can smooth the journey through the challenges of IBS.

IBS can significantly impact daily life and productivity, with some experiencing substantial disruptions. It can cause unexpected flare-ups during work hours, frequent toilet visits that disrupt meetings or social activities, and the need for sudden changes to plans to manage symptoms. These challenges sometimes make it difficult to stick to a regular work routine or fully engage in social events. Managing symptoms effectively is critical, as indicated by research highlighting the extensive impact of IBS on work and personal life. Clear communication and boundary setting are vital to handling these challenges successfully.

The survey highlights the profound effects of IBS on individuals' lives, revealing significant productivity losses and personal distress for some. It emphasises the importance of raising awareness and fostering understanding in various spheres of life, including work, home, and social settings.

Not setting clear boundaries when managing IBS can exacerbate stress and discomfort, affecting overall well-being. Establishing assertive boundaries early, especially in demanding situations, supports effective time management and improves long-term gut health management. Approach each day as it arrives and consistently prioritise communication with your IBS health in mind in all your actions. It is vital to maintain this approach to ensure your well-being remains a priority.

Take the time to teach your close friends, family, and colleagues about IBS. This will help them better understand your condition, making them more empathetic and supportive. It will also create a more caring environment where you feel understood and can manage your symptoms more effectively.

By prioritising clear communication and firm boundaries, individuals with IBS can enhance their quality of life and better manage their symptoms. The practical communication tips discussed would help those with IBS to manage the challenges of IBS with resilience and self-advocacy. This creates a feeling of control and well-being as they continue to work towards better gut health and healing.

Consistency is vital for success. Establishing a daily routine and taking consistent action, no matter how small, promotes progress. Embrace learning and strive for improvement daily, avoiding the trap of perfectionism. Choose satisfaction with achievements while striving for continuous enhancement.

Ultimately, focus on activities that energise rather than drain you, and prioritise moving forward without regrets.

25. Quick tips for managing IBS flare-ups at home

"A very little key will open a very heavy door." — *Charles Dickens*

Managing IBS flare-ups is crucial to lessen discomfort and keep up with daily tasks. Simple adjustments at home can be beneficial. We will explore how everyday items found at home can aid in managing IBS symptoms such as bloating, indigestion, cramps, and more. You can take these practical tips with you for IBS relief wherever you go, highlighting the small changes that are often overlooked but can make a big difference.

Addressing bloating, indigestion, burping, and wind

Handling bloating and gas is a frequent concern for many individuals with IBS.

IBS disrupts regular intestinal contractions, causing irregular bowel movements and symptoms like bloating and diarrhoea. Some individuals with IBS react to specific foods like dairy, gluten, or certain carbohydrates (FODMAPs), which can trigger bloating, gas, and diarrhoea. Emotional stress and anxiety can also impact gut function, contributing to symptoms such as bloating, increased gas, and changes in bowel habits. Changes in the gut microbiome, such as bacterial overgrowth or alterations in bacteria types, can lead to symptoms like bloating and diarrhoea. Managing these symptoms often involves identifying trigger foods and managing stress.

Everyone naturally produces gas, a normal part of the body's functions. However, it can sometimes cause discomfort with gurgling noises, stomach cramps or embarrassment when excessive or smelly. The main signs of gas include burping, passing wind, and feeling bloated. Yet, these symptoms can also be caused by conditions like IBS rather than just excessive gas.

Gas in the digestive system comes from swallowing air and the breakdown of certain foods by bacteria in the large intestine. Eating quickly, chewing gum, sucking on hard candies, and certain foods can increase gas in your digestive system. Some with IBS might be more sensitive and produce more gas than other individuals. This is partly due to foods rich in carbohydrates like beans that often lead to gas. In contrast, fats and proteins generally produce minimal gas.

Cruciferous vegetables such as brussels sprouts and broccoli typically cause gas when eaten in large amounts, unlike kale. Avoiding spicy, fatty or fried foods that take longer to digest, leading to indigestion and gas, could help. Deep frying foods in reused oils, especially if the oil has been reused more than twice, like potato fries, can negatively affect health, particularly concerning bloating and gas. This practice can result in the creation of harmful substances, such as acrylamide, which is known to cause digestive discomfort. Try eating smaller meals and, if required, cook them thoroughly in a pressure cooker to aid digestion. Chew your food slowly to help ease symptoms of bloating and gas. When you do not chew your food properly and swallow it quickly, larger undigested pieces enter your system, leading to various gut issues. Saliva contains digestive enzymes that help break food down into smaller particles, reducing the strain on your digestive system. Chew your food thoroughly to minimise indigestion and prevent bloating.

Hidden salts and carbohydrates in your diet can cause bloating, which can be particularly problematic for individuals with IBS. These hidden ingredients lead to water retention and excessive gas production, making IBS symptoms worse. Drinking warm water can help flush out these excess salts and carbohydrates, reduce bloating, and provide relief. This simple habit supports digestion, hydration, and a healthier gut environment, all crucial for effectively managing IBS. Foods such as processed meats (like bacon and sausage), canned soups, ready meals, condiments (such as ketchup and soy sauce), and packaged snacks (like chips and crackers) are examples of foods with high sodium levels that can worsen bloating and discomfort in individuals with IBS.

It is also ideal to avoid carbonated drinks, as they contain a lot of gas that can lead to bloating and wind for some with IBS. **Try this instead:** when you leave carbonated drinks open for several hours, the gas they contain can escape, reducing the carbonation in the drink. Avoiding carbonated beverages is advisable; instead, opt for green tea, matcha, or non-carbonated drinks to reduce burping and feeling bloated.

Cut back on mints and chewing gum, as some individuals with IBS are more sensitive to the effects of swallowed air, which can accumulate in the digestive tract and cause bloating and flatulence. Sugar-free gums containing artificial sweeteners like sorbitol, mannitol, and xylitol can have a laxative effect when consumed in large amounts. This can worsen bloating in some individuals due to sorbitol intolerance, even with small doses. Sorbitol can cause stomach and bowel symptoms like gas, bloating, and cramps, depending on the quantity ingested (ranging from 5 to 20 grams per day). Consuming more than 20 grams daily can lead to diarrhoea. Effects vary from person to person, and many small factors could contribute to IBS symptoms that we can easily overlook. It is preferable to seek advice from doctors and professionals based on an individual's diagnosis of intolerances, as these can vary. Be mindful of aggressive or prolonged chewing of gum, which can increase air swallowing. Studies on the relationship between gum chewing and bloating have shown mixed results, so consider reducing or eliminating your intake of chewing gum or switching to sugar-free gums with natural sweeteners. **Tip:** instead of chewing gum, occasionally suck on 1-2 cloves per day for better oral and gut health.

Asafoetida, commonly known as Hing in Indian cuisine, reduces gas or wind due to its digestive benefits. It is added in small amounts to dishes, especially those containing beans or lentils, to help minimise the gas these foods can cause. This practice is well-regarded in traditional Indian cooking for easing digestion and reducing flatulence.

Additional home remedies to reduce bloating, indigestion, burping, and wind for those with IBS include:

Take peppermint tea bags or IBS-friendly ginger candies to soothe the digestive tract.

Drink a glass of warm water with a squeeze of lemon juice in the morning.

After eating, chew on a teaspoon of fennel seeds.

Combine one tablespoon of apple cider vinegar in warm water and consume it before meals.

Boil fresh ginger slices in water to make a soothing tea.

By following the dietary tips outlined in the chapter on 'Meal Planning for IBS: Tips and Tricks' and practising exercises such as the Malasana walk and butterfly flaps from the 'Morning and Night Routine for Gut Health and Well-being,' you can ease discomfort caused by excessive gas. Removing foods or drinks from your diet that you suspect may be causing gas is helpful. Gradually reintroduce them individually to identify any triggers and seek medical advice for further guidance.

Adjusting your diet, taking lactase supplements, which are digestive enzymes, and reducing swallowed air are common methods to reduce gas discomfort. Consider other factors, like stress levels, which can contribute to bloating and wind. Pay attention to how different foods affect your body and manage exercise and stress effectively to improve overall well-being.

Handling diarrhoea symptoms

Diarrhoea occurs when you have loose or watery stools more often than usual. It can cause dehydration. Symptoms include feeling exhausted, frequently needing to use the bathroom, stomach pain, nausea, fever, weakness, and loss of appetite. The severity and duration of the symptoms can vary greatly, lasting from days to months.

Natural ways to handle diarrhoea at home:

- Have some plain buttermilk with a pinch of salt to hydrate and calm the stomach.
- Chew or create a paste using 10-15 fresh curry leaves, then mix in 1 teaspoon of honey and consume. Curry leaves have digestive properties, and honey soothes the stomach lining.
- Boil rice in extra water, strain it, and drink the cooled rice water. This can help soothe the digestive system and keep you hydrated.
- Blend a ripe banana with 1 teaspoon of tamarind pulp and a pinch of salt. Consume this mixture twice a day or combine 1/4 teaspoon of nutmeg powder with a ripe banana and eat the mix.
- Drink a cup of strong black tea or 1 cup of fresh pomegranate juice 3 to 4 times a day.
- Consume fresh coconut water to replenish electrolytes and keep the body hydrated.
- Grind 1/4 teaspoon of cardamom seeds into powder. Boil this in diluted tea water. Sweeten with a bit of jaggery powder for flavour and consumption.
- Dry mango seeds in a shaded area for 3-4 days before grinding them into a powder and storing them in a container. Take ½ teaspoon of this powder with either sugar or honey.
- Soak 2-3 teaspoons of coriander seeds overnight in half a cup of water. Mix to a coarse paste thoroughly into a glass of buttermilk before drinking.

You can experiment with the above home remedies slowly and in small quantities, ideally testing one at a time. This approach helps ensure they are suitable and adequate for managing your symptoms. It is essential to monitor how each remedy impacts you and adjust accordingly to find what works for you. Consult a healthcare professional for personalised advice if you have concerns or experience adverse effects. If you experience acute diarrhoea, seek advice from a medical professional and begin oral hydration immediately.

Relief from constipation

Constipation in individuals with IBS can be due to various reasons. The condition disrupts regular bowel movements, slowing down the passage of stool through the digestive system and leading to constipation. Diet is crucial; not consuming enough fibre, drinking too little fluid, or eating foods that trigger symptoms can all contribute. Emotional factors such as stress and anxiety every day in those with IBS also affect how the gut functions and can worsen constipation. Hormonal changes, especially in women, can also affect bowel movements. Managing constipation in IBS involves adjusting your diet, staying hydrated, and managing stress.

Hydration is key in managing constipation. Aim to drink six to eight glasses of about 1.5 to 2 litres of caffeine-free fluids daily. This can help increase the frequency of bowel movements and reduce the need for laxatives. Opt for warm water and a fibre-rich diet, as warm fluids can soften the stool, making it easier to pass. **Tip:** consider enhancing your hydration with electrolytes like fresh coconut water (200-400ml per day) mixed with 1-2 tablespoons of chia seeds for variety. This has been a beneficial part of my daily routine, aiding daily bowel movements. Coconut water contains electrolytes that help the gut absorb nutrients effectively, supporting overall digestive health.

Chia seeds are a natural solution for managing constipation. Rich in soluble fibre called mucilage, they act as a natural laxative by helping food and waste move smoothly through the digestive system. These seeds also absorb water in the digestive tract, forming a gel-like substance that adds volume to stool and supports smoother passage. You can find fresh coconut water on platforms like Amazon click here or check the 'Additional Resources' chapter for the complete link.

Initially, try natural remedies to boost fibre intake and bulk the stool. If symptoms persist, consult a doctor before considering other options, such as laxatives and stool softeners. **Remember**, these natural remedies are designed to bring relief and comfort. **Tip:** gradually increase natural fibre and water intake to avoid worsening symptoms. Limit flaxseed powder intake to 2 tablespoons daily, accompanied by 150 ml of fluid with each tablespoon, and avoid wheat bran. Always remember that it is essential to consult a medical professional or dietitian for accurate diagnosis and dietary guidance.

Based on the USDA Food Composition Database, flax seeds offer a blend of soluble and insoluble fibre, providing 2.8 grams of fibre and 1.9 grams of protein per tablespoon, about 10 grams. Drying roast and grind flax seeds before consuming them is ideal to improve absorption. When eaten whole, they may pass through your system without being fully digested, which reduces their nutritional benefits. Flaxseeds have approximately 8 grams of fibre in about 4 tablespoons, whereas chia seeds contain 10 grams in the same amount. Flaxseeds are richer in insoluble fibre, which is particularly beneficial for relieving constipation. **Bonus tip:** try incorporating fibre-rich exotic fruits like guavas, papayas, and figs into your diet in moderation for added digestive benefits.

Introducing fibre-rich snacks into your diet can be a simple yet effective way to manage constipation. Consider making a trail mix with nuts, seeds, and dried fruits, or including salads, vegetables, and superfoods like Moringa leaves. These choices can help maintain regular bowel movements and improve overall digestive health. You could also try the gentle colon cleanse with fresh neem leaf paste discussed earlier in the chapter 'Lifestyle Practices to Promote a Healthy Microbiome'. It might help some with constipation relief by cleansing the colon.

More ways to relieve constipation at home:

- As discussed in the chapter 'Potential Impact of Body Types on IBS', Triphala might help.
- Kiwifruit contains 2-3% dietary fibre and is thought to have laxative effects. It can significantly improve stool consistency in healthy elderly individuals and those with chronic constipation.
- Psyllium husk adds bulk to stools and makes them easier to pass.
- Applying castor oil around the belly button before bedtime has been personally beneficial.
- Ginger and lemon tea is a comforting beverage.
- Ajwain, or Carom seeds, can be consumed after meals to assist digestion.

- On an empty stomach, have a tablespoon of all-natural extra virgin olive oil with a dash of fresh lemon juice in the morning. Begin with a small amount, such as a teaspoon, for a few days, then gradually increase.

These simple methods also help preserve intestinal flora, which is crucial for overall digestive health. Always seek advice from a healthcare provider before trying any new treatment or remedy, especially if you have underlying health conditions.

Coping with acid reflux and heartburn

Understanding the unique factors that contribute to your IBS symptoms can empower you to effectively manage them. Those with IBS often have a sensitive digestive system, which can cause discomfort and symptoms like acid reflux. Delayed gastric emptying, where food stays in the stomach longer than usual, can pressure the lower oesophageal sphincter, increasing the likelihood of reflux. Heartburn, a symptom of acidity, occurs when stomach acid moves up into the oesophagus, causing a sharp burning sensation in the chest. Stomach ulcers can also develop due to excessive acid secretion. Emotional stress and anxiety every day in IBS can also worsen heartburn symptoms by affecting how the digestive system functions. These factors can differ and interact uniquely for each person, highlighting the importance of identifying and effectively managing triggers.

Eliminate alcohol, spicy and acidic foods, non-vegetarian and oily diets, raw onions, garlic, citrus fruits and non-steroidal anti-inflammatory drugs that may irritate the stomach and worsen acidity problems. Avoid foods that trigger heartburn symptoms, such as hot peppers and chilli. Consume millet as discussed in the chapter 'Meal Planning for IBS: Tips and Tricks' as they are alkaline-forming and promote optimal gut health, helping to maintain a balanced pH and prevent issues like acidity and heartburn, especially beneficial for those with IBS. Giving up smoking can lessen how often and how severe acid reflux is and sometimes even get rid of it altogether.

Avoid lying with a full stomach, as it can worsen acid reflux and heartburn symptoms. To prevent this, refrain from eating within 2-3 hours of bedtime, allowing your stomach ample time to digest food before lying down. Consider intermittent fasting and opt for smaller meals, say 4 to 5 times a day, eaten slowly and chewed thoroughly. This approach can reduce strain on your digestive system. Ensure hydration by drinking ample water. This helps with digestion and keeps you feeling fuller, reducing cravings. **Personal tip:** having the last meal or snack before sunset has been very effective.

These remedies have been tried and tested, offering a safe and effective way to manage your symptoms. **Personal tip:** try the 3-spice tea mix below.

This mix is known as the "Triphala of digestion" in Ayurvedic medicine. It not only reduces indigestion that leads to acid reflux but also soothes menstrual pains, which can impact IBS. The ingredients are:

- Jeera (Cumin) stimulates digestive juices, relieves gas and bloating, and has anti-inflammatory properties.
- Saunf (Fennel): soothes the digestive tract, eases gas, and acts as a mild laxative.
- Ajwain (Caraway) aids digestion, relieves cramps, and has antimicrobial properties.

Whether you have had an occasional late-night meal or indulged in heavy social meals over the weekend, this 3-spice tea mix can help. If you feel sluggish and bloated, consume it on an empty stomach first thing in the morning, particularly if you wake up feeling acidic or gassy. You can also have it 30 minutes before or after your main meals, such as breakfast, lunch, or dinner.

Here is how to prepare the tea using the dry roasting method:

1. Take equal parts of jeera, saunf, and ajwain seeds, readily available in Indian spice aisles at stores.
2. Lightly dry roast them over low heat for a few minutes. Prepare in advance in batches for future use.
3. Gently crush the roasted seeds into coarse pieces.
4. Stir in 1 teaspoon of the mixture into a cup of boiling water.
5. Allow it to steep for 5-10 minutes.
6. Strain and drink warm, preferably before meals every morning, instead of coffee.
7. The dry roasting method explained above saves time.

Another traditional approach involves blending these three spices, roasting them, and creating a post-meal digestive mix. Simply chew on this mixture, which also acts as a potent breath freshener, providing stimulation and a cooling effect for your digestive system, which could help manage heartburn. A similar readymade option found in the Asian aisles in supermarkets is Mukhwas. This traditional Indian mouth freshener contains ingredients that aid digestion and reduce heartburn. Choose the unsweetened version for a healthier option.

The alternative method involves preparing a concoction using the above 3 spices as follows:

To make a daily batch of the concoction, boil the above 3 highly anti-inflammatory spices in 1 litre of water. Let it simmer until the volume reduces to 500 ml. Let it cool in the refrigerator or at room temperature, then transfer it to a glass bottle. Sip on this mixture to help reduce acidity, indigestion, and bloating. Ensure to rule out any allergies and make an informed decision. **Key:** begin with one cup (150 ml), and then gradually increase the amount over the next few days to assess its suitability for you. Nature holds powerful remedies if we use them correctly. It works well for most individuals, though it may not work for some.

Tip: consistency is crucial. Regular consumption of the above 3-spice tea mix, whether as dry roast tea, concoction, or mukhwas, can help prevent and manage indigestion, which can lead to acid reflux and heartburn.

You can try the below to relieve acidity and heartburn at home:

- Chew on a small piece of jaggery after each meal to aid digestion. Jaggery contains potassium and magnesium, which calms your upset stomach. Potassium balances pH levels and promotes stomach lining mucus production to prevent acid build-up and reduce symptoms. Meanwhile, magnesium supports digestion, reducing acidity and other digestive issues.
- After each meal, grind one clove and one cardamom into a powder and use it as a mouth freshener. This will also prevent bad breath.
- Combine cumin tea with other herbs like ginger or fennel for enhanced benefits. Add a touch of fresh lemon or honey to your cumin tea for added flavour. **Top tip:** papaya fruit contains papain, an enzyme that supports protein digestion, potentially reducing acid reflux and heartburn. Consume fully ripe papaya for ideal results.
- Mint leaves help with digestion and provide a cooling effect for your body. Mint leaves offer immediate relief and long-term support against acid reflux, making them a straightforward and effective solution.
- After switching off the stove, limit spicy foods by mixing fresh coconut milk or yoghurt.
- The lactic acid in buttermilk helps to balance stomach acidity and provides a soothing effect. A glass of buttermilk with added black pepper and coriander can quickly ease symptoms of acidity.
- Raising your head and chest higher than your feet while sleeping can prevent and reduce acid reflux and heartburn. Elevate the head of your bed with blocks under the bedposts, or use a foam wedge under the mattress. Avoid using multiple pillows, which are often ineffective and might worsen your symptoms.
- Sleeping on your left side could aid digestion and reduce acid reflux.
- A glass of lukewarm water before breakfast and bedtime can help relieve acidity.
- Avoid tight-fitting belts and opt for loose-fitting clothing to relieve pressure on your stomach.

Adopting the above home remedies that suit your condition and body type allows you to experience natural and effective relief from acidity and heartburn. They offer a holistic approach to managing these IBS symptoms, supporting your well-being with simple and accessible solutions. Take into account your body type according to your dosha, as discussed previously in the chapter 'Potential Impact of Body Types on IBS', to better inform yourself. It is ideal to seek medical advice where needed.

Managing Fatigue and IBS

According to research published in PubMed Central, fatigue commonly accompanies IBS. IBS involves a breakdown in communication between the gut and the brain, with the Vagus nerve playing a crucial role. This nerve, the longest cranial nerve in the body, regulates automatic functions like heartbeat, breathing, and digestion, including stomach acid and bile production.

For the Vagus nerve to function optimally, your body must be relaxed (parasympathetic), supporting digestion (rest and digest). Stress often disrupts this balance, lowering stomach acid and enzyme production. IBS and chronic fatigue syndrome frequently overlap, with both conditions linked to imbalances in the gut microbiome.

Fatigue in IBS can also stem from nutrient deficiencies, such as vitamin B12, which is essential for energy metabolism. Still, it can be depleted by gut bacteria imbalance. Stress worsens symptoms, affecting concentration, sometimes causing joint pain, and hindering nutrient absorption, including vitamins D, E, and A.

In conventional medicine, drugs like antibiotics and pain relievers are used to manage IBS symptoms. However, a holistic approach addressing underlying causes through nutritional therapy and stress management can offer long-term relief. This approach includes assessing:

- Nutrient levels (via blood tests),
- Hormonal imbalance,
- Microbiome health and
- Vagus nerve function through tests.

Make lifestyle adjustments, such as practising mindful eating by eating your last meal before sunset and pairing your complex carbohydrates with fibre-rich vegetables, good-quality protein, fermented foods, probiotics, and healthy fats. Healthy fats, particularly Omega-3s, are essential for brain function, hormonal balance, and managing fatigue. You can get Omega-3s from supplements or fatty fish.

Ensure you plan your week, setting aside time for self-care and adequate rest, which is crucial for body recovery in IBS. Moving your body every hour improves blood circulation, delivering more oxygen and essential nutrients to body tissues, which helps produce energy. Earlier in the chapter 'Morning and Night Routine for Gut Health and Well-being,' we explored how a brief Japanese Radio Taiso exercise can assist in managing fatigue.

Tip: briefly dip your hands in a bowl of ice water for 2 minutes. This can help reduce fatigue in IBS by stimulating the body's cold response and boosting alertness and energy levels. Start with a few seconds and gradually increase. Check with your doctor, especially if you have underlying health conditions, as exposure to cold temperatures is unsuitable.

Practising stress reduction methods such as cold showers, deep breathing, and a brisk walk can provide a quick energy boost. For more details, refer to chapters 'Stress Reduction Work Techniques' and 'Communication Skills with Setting Boundaries at Work and Home'.

If the methods mentioned above are not as effective, taking certain supplements recommended by doctors can also help reduce brain fog, confusion, poor judgment, and difficulty concentrating caused by fatigue often experienced by individuals with IBS. These symptoms are associated with stress, fatigue, and other physical symptoms. Each individual responds differently, so personalised care is essential.

Collaborate with a dietitian to effectively manage your IBS symptoms that improve the long-term health of your gut microbiome.

CHAPTER RECAP:

Managing IBS involves making simple changes at home to tackle various symptoms. Bloating, indigestion, and wind often flare up due to certain foods, hormonal imbalances, lifestyle, underlying health conditions and stress.

Lifestyle adjustments like regular exercise and relaxation techniques can reduce stress, which worsens IBS symptoms. Managing stress is essential, so use relaxation techniques like deep breathing or yoga.

Eating mindfully and avoiding triggers like spicy and fatty foods can help improve digestion. Natural remedies such as peppermint tea and asafoetida can calm the stomach and reduce excessive gas. Ensure your diet is varied, avoid eating due to emotions, and avoid alcohol and smoking for a healthy gut microbiome that contributes to better symptom management. Plan your meals ahead so they are nutritious, have plenty of fibre (adults aiming for 30 grams per day), contain healthy fats, and have enough water. Food variety is essential for nourishing gut microbes. Regular exercise and sufficient sleep are vital for your overall well-being.

For diarrhoea, remedies like coconut water, curry leaves with honey, rice water, and black tea provide hydration and relief.

Constipation can be eased by drinking enough warm fluids, eating foods high in fibre, and trying natural remedies such as Triphala and ginger tea. Applying castor oil around the belly button before bedtime has personally helped me. In addition, drinking warm water with apple cider vinegar in the morning on an empty stomach helped with regular bowel movements. Keep in mind that results may vary for each person.

Managing acid reflux and heartburn involves avoiding triggers and using remedies like a 3-spice tea mix, jaggery, and sleeping with your head elevated.

Managing fatigue includes holistic approaches to addressing stress and nutrient deficiencies and improving Vagus nerve function through lifestyle changes, supplements, and personalised care. For example, you could do a short Japanese Radio Taiso exercise or a brisk walk to boost energy. Try brief cold water immersions or cold showers to boost your energy levels quickly. Start slowly and talk to your doctor if you are unsure about exposure to freezing temperatures or have underlying health conditions that could worsen IBS symptoms.

When trying home remedies for IBS flare-ups, it is ideal to choose wisely and test them one at a time to see what works for you. IBS can differ significantly from person to person, which can make you feel like your concerns are not being heard. Always seek advice from your doctor for further guidance. Listen to your body and adjust your habits and routines to support your gut health.

Looking Ahead: Research and Future Directions

"Happiness often sneaks in through a door you didn't know you left open." — John Barrymore

This chapter will explore why a diverse microbiome is crucial for keeping our gut healthy and maintaining overall well-being. We will also discuss recent breakthroughs in microbiome science that are helping to develop new and alternative treatments for IBS. These advancements aim to manage IBS more effectively and improve the quality of life for those with it.

26. Understanding the role of Microbiome diversity in gut health

"For all evils there are two remedies - time and silence." — Alexandre Dumas

We will discuss why microbiome diversity is crucial for maintaining gut health and overall well-being.

Role of the gut microbiome in health

The gut microbiome is a continuously evolving field of study, with scientists consistently uncovering new insights into how it affects human health and disease. Understanding how the gut microbiome functions is vital for developing tailored approaches to prevent and treat various health conditions, such as IBS, IBD, obesity, allergies, and even mental health disorders like depression and anxiety. Studying microbiome diversity helps spot patterns that relate to different health problems.

The diverse community of microorganisms that live in the human gut has a wide range of metabolic abilities that complement the functions of enzymes in the liver and stomach lining. These microbes are essential for breaking down food and influencing how nutrients affect our health. Researchers are particularly interested in identifying specific microorganisms involved in various metabolic processes, including breaking down dietary carbohydrates into short-chain fatty acids and gases, processing proteins, and metabolising plant polyphenols, bile acids, and vitamins. Understanding these microbial pathways is vital to uncovering their impact on human metabolism and overall health.

Scientists are discovering more about how these microbes impact digestion, the immune system, and overall health. The microbiome supports various digestive functions, creating a solid community that can adjust to changes in your lifestyle, such as shifts in diet, stress levels, and medications. This adaptability helps maintain gut health and overall well-being.

Importance of microbiome diversity

Recent advancements highlight the importance of microbiome diversity in promoting efficient digestion, nutrient absorption, and stable mood regulation. A balanced microbiome produces essential vitamins and breaks down dietary fibres, contributing to overall health.

Factors that influence microbiome diversity

Diet:
As previously discussed, it is beneficial to consume a variety of foods, such as fibre-rich foods, fruits, vegetables, and fermented foods, to support microbiome diversity. The more fibre you include in your diet, the more fuel your gut microbiome has to work with, which can lead to better psychological health.

The researchers discovered that individuals who transitioned to the Mediterranean diet and adhered to it consistently experienced beneficial alterations in their gut microbiome. These changes were associated with several health improvements, such as reduced frailty risk and improved cognitive function. Moreover, the study observed decreased blood markers that typically indicate chronic inflammation. **Personal tip:** it is ideal to steer clear of foods that trigger your IBS and instead embrace a diverse global diet.

Managing IBS symptoms often involves dietary interventions like the low FODMAP diet, which restricts fermentable carbohydrates. Clinical studies support the efficacy of this diet in reducing IBS symptoms. However, its impact on gut microbiome composition varies among individuals. Recent research suggests that microbiome activity and composition differences may influence individual responses to the low FODMAP diet, highlighting the potential for personalised approaches in managing IBS.

Including various colourful fruits and vegetables in your diet, known as "eating the rainbow," helps diversify your gut microbiome in several ways. Different coloured foods contain various fibre, vitamins, minerals, and antioxidants that nourish and enrich the gut bacteria. For example, fibre-rich foods like leafy greens and berries provide prebiotics that support the growth of beneficial bacteria in the gut. Antioxidants in colourful vegetables and fruits help reduce inflammation and maintain a balanced microbial community, supporting overall gut health. Including these foods in your diet can promote better health and a diverse gut microbiome, essential for effective digestion, nutrient absorption, and overall well-being.

Foods rich in polyphenols, like dark chocolate, can also support microbiome diversity. Cocoa and it's products are known for their health benefits. The polyphenolic profile of cocoa can vary based on the type of cocoa, where it is grown, and how it is processed. The health effects and availability of cocoa polyphenols depend on their structure and concentration, individual factors and interactions with other nutrients in food. These polyphenols reach the colon and are broken down by gut bacteria into more minor compounds, which then influence the microbial population in the gut. Studies have shown that cocoa has prebiotic effects, encouraging the growth of beneficial bacteria like Lactobacillus and Bifidobacterium while reducing harmful ones like certain Clostridium species. Cocoa's health benefits are primarily due to its antioxidant and anti-inflammatory properties. However, the precise mechanisms behind these benefits still need to be fully understood. More research is required to explore the interactions between cocoa polyphenols and gut bacteria and their overall impact on health.

Environment:

Research into the connections between the environment, gut microbiota, and inflammation is a rapidly evolving field. Its goal is to investigate how traditional diets and local soil conditions influence the diversity of gut microbes through various transmission routes. Understanding how environmental microbes are transmitted, whether through breathing, eating, or skin contact, is crucial for guiding further research. Urbanisation and soil degradation likely impact the composition of gut microbes, potentially increasing bacteria associated with dysbiosis, such as Proteobacteria. Standardising methods for collecting, extracting, and preparing samples, alongside detailed metadata reporting and robust analysis platforms, is crucial for advancing this research.

Key challenges include developing reliable methods to quantify the richness and diversity of microbes in different environments and understanding how landscape features and community biodiversity influence microbiota composition. Enhancing tools for collecting, storing, and analysing large datasets on interactions between hosts, microbiomes, and environments is also essential. Current limitations in sample handling, storage, and reporting hinder comparing studies and fully understanding demographic factors. Collaborative efforts, potentially integrating with initiatives like the NIH Human Microbiome Project, could improve understanding of how environmental factors shape gut microbiota and their implications for human health.

Professor Jack Gilbert, a distinguished microbiome scientist at the University of California San Diego and author of "Dirt Is Good," has received accolades for his research in microbiology. His research has shown that since the gut microbiome is established early in life, allowing young children to play in soil and with pets can help counteract the adverse effects of modern lifestyles on their gut health. This early exposure helps establish a healthier and more varied community of microorganisms in the gut, which is vital for managing conditions like IBS. A diverse microbiome supports better immune function, reduces inflammation, and improves digestion, all of which contribute to reducing symptoms of IBS. Encouraging such exposure from an early age may offer long-term benefits for gut health, potentially lowering the risk of developing gut-related disorders later in life.

Exercise:

A study across 1,044 participants revealed that regular exercise leads to a notable increase in gut microbiota diversity among adults. Regular exercise showed higher levels of Firmicutes bacteria and lower levels of Bacteroidetes than those who did not exercise regularly. Researchers must consider demographic factors and exercise intensity, as women and older adults may respond differently. To fully understand the long-term effects of exercise on gut microbiota, more well-designed studies of extended duration and larger number of participants are required.

Sleep:
Metabolism refers to the body's essential chemical processes that sustain life, encompassing three main functions: converting food into energy for cellular activities, building proteins, lipids, nucleic acids, and carbohydrates, and eliminating metabolic waste. A group of metabolic issues, including high blood pressure, central obesity, insulin resistance, and atherogenic dyslipidemia, collectively known as metabolic syndrome, is associated with sleep duration. Research suggests a U-shaped relationship where 7 hours of sleep per night is optimal. Sleeping less or more than 7 hours increases the risk of metabolic syndrome, including obesity, type 2 diabetes, and hypertension. Those who sleep 5 hours or 9 hours also face similarly heightened risks compared to those who sleep 7 hours.

Stress:
Pressure is a natural reaction to difficult circumstances. Still, prolonged exposure can have lasting effects that disrupt the balance of gut bacteria. Research shows that chronic stress alters the composition of gut microbes, reducing beneficial bacteria and increasing harmful ones. This imbalance is linked to conditions like IBS, IBD, and even depression, all of which can worsen with stress. A nutritious diet, consistent physical activity, and stress-reducing practices help maintain a healthy gut microbiome. Understanding this connection allows you to actively support both gut health and overall well-being.

Ageing:
The relationship between gut microbiota (GM), ageing, and longevity has become increasingly clear in recent years, highlighting its significant impact on how we age. Various factors affect the diversity of GM among individuals, including unique biological traits, lifestyle habits affecting both mind and body, environmental factors, and age itself. Comparisons between centenarians and younger older adults have revealed differences in the types of microbes present in their guts, suggesting that GM could be a promising target for therapies aimed at promoting healthy ageing.

Although there are limitations to current research, many studies have examined the potential benefits of probiotics, prebiotics, and symbiotic products that combine probiotics and prebiotics to support gut health, physical activity, and the Mediterranean diet in modifying GM composition. These interventions have shown promise in potentially delaying the onset of ageing-related issues. They may improve colon health, bolster immune responses, regulate cholestrol levels in blood, enhance cognitive function and muscle strength, while also reducing inflammation, oxidative stress, and the presence of harmful bacteria. Given the significant influence of GM on the ageing process, further in-depth research is required to develop effective therapeutic strategies that can help individuals live longer, healthier lives through better management of their gut health.

Genetics:
Genetics contribute substantially to each person's microbiome's unique composition and diversity. Variations in genetic makeup influence which microorganisms thrive in different individuals, shaping their microbial communities. These genetic differences can determine how effectively the microbiome performs essential functions such as nutrient metabolism, immune system modulation, and protection against diseases. Researchers are increasingly exploring these genetic factors to better grasp their impact on health and illness, aiming to develop personalised strategies that take into account microbiome diversity for improved well-being.

Medications:
Saliva samples were collected from 846 women and 368 men aged 35–69 years participating in the Atlantic Partnership for Tomorrow's Health (PATH), a Canadian population cohort. These samples underwent analysis to investigate variations in microbial community structures among non-users of medications, those using a single drug, and those using multiple drugs. The study focused on the effects of three commonly prescribed medications: thyroid hormones, statins, and proton pump inhibitors (PPIs). It found that the oral microbiome is relatively consistent among individuals without primary chronic conditions who take commonly prescribed medications, although there were minor changes in a few types of bacteria. It showed that these medications have little impact on the variety of microbes in saliva and cause only slight differences in the numbers of specific bacterial groups. This indicates that these

medications do not significantly alter the composition of the saliva microbiome in individuals who do not have primary chronic conditions.

This analysis provided a foundation for future research that can look into specific medication types, dosages, durations, and methods of administration. The oral microbiome holds promise as a potential tool for monitoring health status, predicting future disease risks, or anticipating treatment outcomes. However, further investigation is crucial to understand how different diseases and their corresponding treatments influence the oral microbiome. Future studies are essential to examine individuals with IBS both before and after starting specific medications, with adequate controls in large cohorts.

Avoiding antibiotics, except when prescribed by a doctor, can also aid in maintaining a healthy balance of microbes in the gut. Early attention to gut health can prevent future microbiome-related issues. Diagnostic tests can identify any changes that may require intervention.

Technological advances in microbiome research

Scientists use advanced technology to study the types and functions of gut microbes, enabling them to identify specific bacteria and understand their interactions within the gut. This involves carefully storing and processing stool samples to extract microbial DNA and perform metagenomic analysis, which provides insights into the composition and abundance of gut bacteria.

Genetic variability and microbiome composition

Identifying the types of bacteria in stool samples requires a detailed examination of genetic fragments, which can be intricate due to bacterial DNA swapping and evolution. This process is rapid, akin to your pet dog seeming like a different animal by day's end. Researchers classify bacteria as the same species if their genome sequences are 95% similar or more. In the human gut microbiome, most bacteria belong to two main groups known as Bacteroides and Firmicutes, each encompassing hundreds of species. Despite progress in identifying known species, a significant portion of the microbiome remains unidentified.

Microbiota's impact on gastrointestinal health

Comparative studies between animals without any germs and those with normal bacteria in their bodies, along with research using samples of human faeces, provide valuable information on how the bacteria in the body help process nutrients from food and affect overall health. Observational research comparing healthy individuals with those with IBS shows that gut microbiota significantly influences gastrointestinal diseases such as IBD, IBS, colon cancer, and antibiotic-associated diarrhea. Emerging evidence also links the microbiota to conditions like obesity and diabetes.

Dysbiosis and gut-related disorders

Ongoing investigation into the complexity of the microbiome and its potential manipulation for improving health outcomes highlights its significance in medical research. Recent studies demonstrate that individuals with IBS often exhibit distinct gut bacteria patterns, which may exacerbate symptoms. IBS is associated with an increase in certain bacteria like Firmicutes, including Ruminococcus, Clostridium, and Dorea, and a decrease in beneficial microbes such as Bifidobacterium and Faecalibacterium spp. Harmful bacteria from the Proteobacteria phylum, such as Enterobacteriaceae and Lactobacillaceae families and Bacteroides genus, have also been noted in individuals with IBS. This is possibly linked to past infections or changes in the gut environment, producing by-products that contribute to symptoms like abdominal pain, bloating, and diarrhoea. Studies exploring probiotics containing Bifidobacterium have shown promise in reducing IBS symptoms compared to products containing Lactobacillus alone.

Dysbiosis, an imbalance in gut bacterial communities, triggers immune system activation and mild inflammation. This is backed by compelling evidence of an increased IBS risk following acute gastroenteritis, characterised by rapid stomach and intestinal inflammation. The higher chance of getting IBS after an infection is not tied to one type of infection, such as bacteria, viruses, or parasites. It shows that different infections can activate the immune system in individuals with certain factors that include genetic predispositions, previous health conditions, or environmental influences.

Emerging insights into microbiome patterns

Recent research utilising advanced sequencing and machine learning identifies specific microbiome patterns linked to severe forms of IBS. Studies also reveal reduced diversity and stability in the gut microbiota of those with IBS. Furthermore, changes in the fungal community (mycobiome) among individuals with IBS may contribute to heightened gut sensitivity.

Future directions in microbiome research

The diverse metabolic capabilities of gut microorganisms complement liver and gut lining enzymes, supporting food digestion and nutrient utilisation. Substantial variability in microbiome composition between individuals exists, with even identical twins sharing only 37% of the same gut microbes. Genetic factors are implicated in identifying the bacteria that thrive in each individual's gut.

Scientists are working towards creating personalised ways to manage and prevent gut-related diseases by exploring and supporting microbiome diversity. This could greatly improve the lives of many.

Ongoing research increasingly shows the connection between gut dysbiosis and IBS. Exploring this connection might pave the way for innovative diagnosing and managing IBS strategies.

CHAPTER RECAP:

The importance of a diverse microbiome in gut health is vital for overall well-being.The study of the gut microbiome is always evolving, with scientists finding new insights into how it affects our health and diseases. This microbiome plays a vital role in conditions like IBS, obesity, allergies, and mental health issues. By examining the diversity in our microbiome, researchers can identify patterns that relate to various health problems and develop tailored ways to prevent and treat these issues.

The diverse microorganisms in our gut have a wide range of abilities that help with functions normally performed by enzymes in the liver and gut lining. These microbes are essential for breaking down food and influencing how nutrients affect our health. They process carbohydrates, proteins, plant compounds, bile acids, and vitamins. Understanding these processes is crucial to revealing how they impact our metabolism and overall health.

Having a diverse microbiome is important for good digestion, nutrient absorption, and stable mood regulation. A balanced microbiome helps produce essential vitamins and break down dietary fibres, which contributes to our health. Factors such as diet, environment, exercise, sleep, stress, ageing, genetics, and medications could influence microbiome diversity.

Eat a variety of global foods, including fibre-rich fruits and vegetables and fermented foods, to support microbiome diversity. The more fibre you consume, the more fuel your gut microbiome gets, which can improve your mental health.

New technologies allow scientists to study gut microbes and their functions in more detail. Techniques like metagenomic analysis give insights into the composition and abundance of gut bacteria, helping researchers better understand and treat different health conditions. Identifying bacteria in stool samples involves looking at genetic fragments, which can be complex due to changes in bacterial DNA. Most gut bacteria belong to two main groups, Bacteroides and Firmicutes, but many species are still unknown.

The gut microbiota exerts a substantial influence on gastrointestinal health, affecting diseases like IBD and IBS and conditions such as obesity and diabetes. An imbalance in the gut bacteria, known as dysbiosis, may cause different health problems by triggering the immune system and inflammation, increasing the risk of IBS. Recent research using advanced techniques has identified specific microbiome patterns linked to severe IBS, showing reduced diversity and stability in the gut microbiota of individuals with IBS.

Researchers are developing personalised treatments based on microbiome diversity to better manage gut-related diseases. Exploring the connection between gut dysbiosis and IBS may open up novel methods for diagnosing and managing IBS. By discussing and supporting microbiome diversity, scientists hope to create ways to manage and prevent diseases related to gut problems, which could significantly improve many individuals' lives. Ongoing research continues to show the importance of a diverse gut microbiome for overall health and well-being.

27. Latest Advances in Microbiome Science and IBS Treatments

"Don't try to add more years to your life. Better add more life to your years." — Blaise Pascal

During the 2010s, interest in the gut microbiome surged in life sciences research and industry, leading Forbes to name it "The Decade of the Microbiome." This rise was primarily driven by initiatives like the National Institutes of Health's "The Human Microbiome Project" and the MetaHIT project funded by the European Union. The International Human Microbiome Consortium was established in 2005 to explore how the microbiome influences human health and disease. These initiatives aim to use this understanding to prevent and treat diseases, marking significant progress in the field.

Recent advancements in microbiome science are changing how we understand and treat IBS. Researchers are discovering how various gut microbes impact our health and well-being. These new insights are leading to better treatments that bring hope and relief to those with IBS. By looking into these advances, we see how the gut and brain are connected and learn about effective ways to manage IBS, helping those affected to have a better quality of life.

Latest breakthroughs in microbiome science that are leading to new and better treatments for IBS include:

Faecal microbiota transplantation

Faecal Microbiota Transplantation (FMT) is being explored for its potential to restore gut microbiota balance in individuals with IBS, particularly in difficult-to-treat or managed cases. Although research is in its early stages, FMT has shown promise in reducing IBS symptoms by reintroducing healthy microbial communities to the gut.

FMT involves transferring stool from a healthy donor into the gut of someone with IBS. The goal is to restore a healthy balance of gut bacteria. This procedure prepares the donor stool by filtering and diluting it, then administers it to the recipient through capsules, enemas, or colonoscopy.

For those with IBS, FMT shows promise because it can help reset the gut microbiota, which is often out of balance. This imbalance can cause symptoms like stomach pain, bloating, and irregular bowel movements. By introducing healthy bacteria from a donor, FMT aims to improve these symptoms and restore normal gut function.

Research into FMT for IBS is ongoing, but early studies suggest it could provide hope for those who have not found relief with other treatments. It offers a new way to treat IBS by addressing the underlying cause of gut imbalance rather than just managing symptoms.

Microbiome modulators

Microbiome modulators such as probiotics, prebiotics, and synbiotics are treatments to improve gut health for those with IBS. Probiotics are good bacteria and yeasts that help restore a healthy balance in the gut. Prebiotics are fibres that feed these helpful bacteria, supporting their growth and activity. Synbiotics combine both probiotics and prebiotics to enhance their effectiveness.

For those with IBS, these therapies target symptoms like stomach pain, bloating, and irregular bowel movements by promoting a healthier gut environment. By restoring the variety and function of gut microbes, microbiome modulators offer a personalised approach to managing IBS symptoms based on each person's unique gut health.

These treatments offer hope for improving daily life for individuals with IBS by potentially reducing how often and severely symptoms occur. They represent a promising path for future therapies that address the root causes of IBS.

Research into the human gut microbiome has become a key focus in biology and medicine, offering valuable insights into how our microbial partners impact health and disease. There is growing interest in altering the microbiome to prevent or treat illnesses, leading to the development of various strategies. However, progress is slowed by uncertainties about the precise role of the microbiome in different conditions, variations in how diseases manifest among individuals, and challenges in formulating and delivering potential therapies. These advancements are essential to integrate microbiota modulation into mainstream medical practices.

Metagenomics and metabolomics

Metagenomics and metabolomics are scientific methods used to study the gut and body chemicals to learn more about IBS. Metagenomics focuses on the genetic material of gut microbes, while metabolomics examines various chemical substances in the body. By studying gut bacteria and substances in faeces and blood, researchers have discovered differences in individuals with IBS compared to healthy individuals. These differences include changes in how the body processes energy and how chemicals in the brain and gut communicate.

For those with IBS, these findings offer hope. Metabolomics has identified specific substances, like THDOC in the blood linked to depression, that show significant differences between individuals with and without IBS. This could lead to improved methods for diagnosing IBS and understanding its links to conditions like depression. Understanding these chemical changes might also lead to new treatments, such as adjusting diets or developing targeted therapies.

These studies improve our understanding of how gut bacteria and body chemistry influence IBS. They offer the potential for developing personalised treatments that could enhance the lives of those with IBS by addressing specific symptoms such as stomach pain, diarrhoea, or constipation. This foundational research is relevant not only to IBS but also to a range of other conditions, including metabolic syndrome, liver diseases, and IBD. It creates new avenues for better understanding and managing IBS in the future.

Microbial signaling pathways

Understanding how diet, gut microbes, and the body interact in IBS remains to be seen, relying mainly on symptoms for diagnosis and treatment outcomes. New research suggests focusing on metabolite variations from both the host and microbes could offer vital insights into IBS. Metabolites are small molecules that produce energy formed during the body's metabolic processes. They are essential because they provide clues about our health, how diseases progress, and the impacts of treatments like changes in diet or medications. Studying metabolites helps scientists and healthcare experts understand how our bodies work and respond to various factors, which is vital for developing effective treatments and improving overall health.

The study explored two main themes: critical metabolites linked to IBS and dietary interventions to reduce symptoms and severity of IBS. While clinical studies on reducing IBS symptoms through diet are increasing, further investigation into the underlying mechanisms of these interventions is required.

The microbiome's role in functional gastrointestinal disorders (FGDs) is well-supported. However, whether or not it causes or correlates with IBS requires further study. Investigating microbially produced metabolites and their impact on gut health and beyond is crucial. These metabolites indicate specific biological processes, offering insights into how diet affects IBS symptoms. Changes in diet affect FGD severity, but understanding why FGDs develop and reducing or proactively preventing them globally requires more than measuring colonic transit time alone.

Colonic transit time refers to how long it takes for food to move through the colon, from when it enters until it leaves the body as stool. Typically, this process takes between 24 to 72 hours. Transit times outside this range, less than 24 hours (fast) or more than 72 hours (slow), are considered abnormal. Changes in colonic transit time can lead to symptoms such as constipation or diarrhoea, which are often prevalent in conditions like IBS.

Thorough studies that combine diet changes with analysis of gut bacteria and metabolites could lead to better dietary advice for effectively reducing IBS symptoms.

Personalised medicine approaches

Using advanced technologies like genomics, transcriptomics, and proteomics to tailor treatment plans based on each person's gut microbiome is an exciting medical frontier. Genomics studies all the genes in an organism to understand health. Transcriptomics studies the RNA molecules to understand gene expression. Proteomics studies the proteins to understand their functions.

By understanding and targeting each person's unique microbial makeup, personalised medicine offers hope for more accurate and effective treatments for conditions like IBS. Integrating and using omics data involves studying genetics, RNA, and protein information to better understand how diseases develop and progress.

The success of this approach depends on shifting from a narrow focus to a broader perspective, sharing data across different fields, and supporting research initiatives. The need to apply biomedical knowledge to improve patient care is improving. These advances will lead to better strategies for preventing, diagnosing, monitoring, and treating diseases, possibly making precision medicine a realistic goal for the future.

Advanced bioinformatics tools, including machine learning and artificial intelligence

Bioinformatics tools are software and methods for studying biological data, like DNA sequences and protein structures. They help researchers make sense of large amounts of biological information by analysing patterns and relationships. On the other hand, machine learning is a type of artificial intelligence where computers learn from data to make decisions or predictions without explicit instructions. In bioinformatics, machine learning can predict biological outcomes or classify data patterns using predictive models. Both are essential in biological research, with bioinformatics tools focusing on data analysis and interpretation. At the same time, machine learning helps make predictions based on biological data.

Recent advances in machine learning, sequencing technologies, and bioinformatics pipelines have transformed the use of gut microbiome knowledge to improve patient health outcomes. Sequencing technologies are essential for reading and analysing genetic information, focusing on the order of DNA bases in genomes to understand biological functions and applications. The variety of sequencing and bioinformatics methods available can produce varied results, highlighting the need for a systematic approach. This includes carefully designing studies, selecting algorithms, and rigorously documenting each step using tools like BioCompute Objects.

BioCompute Objects standardise and document processes in bioinformatics studies, helping researchers and clinicians track every analysis step. They ensure reliable results that are easily interpretable and shareable among professionals. Despite the availability of software tools for multi-omics research in clinical settings, their outputs often need more user-friendly reports for clinicians and require technical expertise to maintain result validity.

Future advancements in multi-omics and machine learning should take a collaborative approach to develop intuitive reporting mechanisms that facilitate evidence-based clinical decision-making. This cooperative effort has the potential to fully exploit multi-omics approaches in understanding the role of the gut microbiome and advancing precision medicine. Overcoming these challenges is crucial to realising this vision and benefiting a broader community.

Recent technological advancements indicate ongoing growth in the years ahead. There are concerns about increasing human reliance on machines, potentially reducing our ability to perform tasks independently. However, it is essential to acknowledge that technology enhances efficiency and maintains high standards, particularly in medical fields. Balancing dependence on technology with personal development remains crucial. When used appropriately, artificial intelligence (AI) systems offer significant benefits. In summary, diagnosing and treating IBS remains challenging. Yet, advancements in AI may provide answers as technology continues to progress.

Postbiotics

Postbiotics are the metabolic products created by probiotic bacteria. They are being studied for their potential to improve gut health and reduce symptoms of IBS. Unlike probiotics, which are live microorganisms that can colonise the body over time, postbiotics are consumed directly and lose potency more quickly.

Research suggests that postbiotics could offer a new approach to treating IBS by:

- Protecting against harmful bacteria through actions like disrupting biofilms and producing antimicrobial substances.
- Strengthening the gut's protective barrier by enhancing protein expression and forming a protective layer.
- Influencing the immune system in various ways, such as through metabolites and components of bacterial cell structures.

Understanding and using the benefits of postbiotics may lead to more effective treatments for IBS, providing hope for individuals seeking relief from symptoms like stomach pain, diarrhoea, wind, and constipation. Further research is required to optimise their use and explore potential combinations with probiotics for enhanced therapeutic effects.

Microbial signatures

Scientists use advanced methods to identify specific microbial signatures linked to different types of IBS. By analysing the unique microbial profiles in the gut, they can develop targeted therapies to help those with IBS.

Microbial signatures are unique patterns of bacteria found in various body parts. The study looked at different types of gastrointestinal (GI) cancers. They found that microbial profiles vary significantly between the upper and lower GI tracts. They discovered that certain bacteria are linked to specific areas and stages of cancer, which helps to anticipate how the disease will develop and its outcome.

This research shows that by studying the microbial community in human tissues using genome sequencing data, scientists can identify important bacterial species that may influence health and disease. Genome sequencing involves reading the entire genetic code of an organism. It allows scientists to understand the order of DNA bases, which make up the genes of living things. By examining this complete genetic information, researchers can gain insights into how organisms function, identify genetic mutations, and explore the links between genetics and diseases. This technology is crucial for advancing personalised medicine and understanding various health conditions. The genome sequencing approach can also be applied to IBS, where understanding these microbial signatures can lead to better treatments.

For those with IBS, this means hope for the future. Targeting specific bacteria in the gut might reduce IBS symptoms. This personalised approach to medicine could enhance the quality of life for many of those with IBS, offering more effective and tailored treatments.

Butyrate and microbial metabolites

Research into butyrate and other microbial metabolites focuses on keeping the gut lining healthy and controlling immune responses in IBS. These compounds could be vital to creating new treatments.

The interaction between gut bacteria and the body in IBS is still being explored. It is tricky to agree on how specific metabolites from gut bacteria relate to different types of IBS. New studies suggest that instead of just looking at symptoms, we need to understand how changes in these metabolites affect IBS.

A study pointed out significant variations in metabolites among individuals with IBS. Metabolites are small molecules that play critical roles in various biological processes within the body, making them essential components. They found that the types and amounts of these crucial metabolites vary between IBS subtypes like IBS-C and IBS-D. This discovery could help diagnose and treat different types of IBS. Metabolites like bile acids, short-chain fatty acids (SCFAs), vitamins, amino acids, serotonin (5-HT), and hypoxanthine are produced by bacteria or diet. Changes in these metabolite levels give us clues about their roles in IBS symptoms.

For example, SCFAs can influence how fast the bowel moves, which is essential for IBS-D. Low levels of hypoxanthine might be linked to problems with energy and colon repair. This suggests that different IBS subtypes may have unique metabolic issues needing tailored treatments.

Metabolites from gut bacteria play a role in IBS severity. Future research should include clinical studies to better understand these interactions. Adding butyrate might help improve bowel movement speed, and further study on its effects on those with IBS is required. To make real progress, combining these treatments with a detailed gut microbiota analysis is needed. This approach would help researchers and scientists understand IBS better and develop targeted therapies.

Ongoing research and careful analysis are crucial for providing safe and effective treatments for IBS, ensuring that recommendations for metabolite-based therapies lead to lasting benefits without causing long-term problems.

Gut microbiota-targeted drugs

New treatments focusing on the gut microbiota are being explored to help manage IBS symptoms. These treatments aim to rebalance the gut bacteria and improve overall gut health. Research indicates that differences in gut bacteria composition are linked to mental health issues, suggesting that adjusting this balance with psychiatric drugs could benefit both mental and digestive health.

Probiotics, known as psychobiotics, are another promising area of study. Clinical trials have demonstrated that these live bacteria positively affect mental health when taken sufficiently. For example, probiotics containing Lactobacillus and Bifidobacterium strains have been shown to improve symptoms in psychiatric individuals, such as reducing insulin resistance and inflammation. These must be administered through medical advice only.

Moreover, the study revealed that combining medications with antipsychotic medications may promote the growth of beneficial bacteria like Akkermansia muciniphila, positively affecting metabolism and insulin sensitivity (Depommier et al., 2019). This dual approach can enhance treatment outcomes while managing potential gut-related side effects.

In summary, these advancements in gut microbiota-targeted therapies offer hope for individuals with IBS by potentially providing more effective and personalised treatments. As research continues and clinical trials progress, understanding the interactions between drugs and the microbiota will be crucial in optimising therapy and minimising complications. This could significantly improve the quality of life for individuals with IBS and related conditions.

Neurobiological mechanisms

Studying how the nervous and immune systems work together in individuals with IBS is vital for understanding how the condition develops and progresses. This research aims to create new treatments that tackle IBS's physical and emotional aspects. SSRIs refer to Selective serotonin reuptake inhibitors (SSRIs) that are sometimes prescribed to help manage symptoms related to the gut and mental health.

The research indicates that while SSRIs and therapies aimed at improving bowel movements benefit specific individuals, they advocate for a comprehensive treatment strategy. This approach includes medicines, behaviour changes, and dietary adjustments. Each person with IBS would respond differently to treatments, depending on their main bowel habits, the severity of gut and mental symptoms, and possible changes in gut bacteria.

The study suggests that there are shared factors (pathophysiological) between IBS and other pain or psychiatric conditions. Pathophysiological factors are abnormalities or dysfunctions that affect the body's work, often contributing to disease or health conditions. These factors may involve genetic predispositions and environmental influences, particularly during childhood, which shape how IBS symptoms manifest. This new understanding challenges the idea of treating IBS with a single approach. It supports using personalised strategies that combine treatments tailored to each person's unique situation.

Gut-brain axis interventions

Research into treatments that affect how the gut and brain communicate to ease IBS symptoms shows promising results. These treatments aim to regulate brain signals and neurotransmitters, offering hope for significant relief for those with IBS. Currently, managing IBS is challenging because existing medications may not work well on their own. Many individuals with IBS have imbalances in their gut bacteria, which are closely linked to when their symptoms start and how severe they are. While probiotics have shown some promise in treating IBS, researchers do not fully understand how they work.

Those with IBS often have symptoms related to problems with neurotransmitters, which affect the gut environment. Growing evidence shows that gut bacteria and neurotransmitters communicate in both directions, influencing blood flow, nutrient absorption, immunity, and movement to keep the gut healthy. A better understanding of this connection could reveal new ways to treat IBS. However, the gut is controlled by many different systems, including hormones from within the gastrointestinal tract and brain, which can change how neurotransmitters affect the gut. Most research has focused on serotonin and GABA, with less attention on histamine and dopamine, suggesting a need for more study on these neurotransmitters in gut diseases. Serotonin and GABA are substances in the brain that influence mood and relaxation. Gut microbes can create neurotransmitters and play a role in regulating them along the gut-brain axis.

Exploring how gut bacteria affect neurotransmitter signals could lead to innovative treatments. Animal studies support this idea, but researchers need more clinical trials to confirm these findings in humans. The research lays the groundwork for further research into how neurotransmitters and gut bacteria interact in IBS, offering hope for better treatments in the future.

Functional magnetic resonance imaging is a brain imaging technique that accurately measures changes in brain activity. Using special brain scans to study individuals with IBS is very important. For example, it can detect how different brain parts respond when a person experiences stomach discomfort or feels stressed. By understanding this better, doctors can create more effective treatments. With better knowledge, doctors can also offer personalised treatment plans, making it easier for each person to manage their symptoms and live a more normal life. This progress brings new hope and reassurance to those coping with IBS.

Epigenetic modifications

Epigenetics studies gene changes and how they are controlled in individuals with IBS. This can help find markers and treatments tailored to each person. It could lead to better ways to manage IBS symptoms, such as stomach discomfort and digestive issues, to name a few. By closely examining how stress, genetics, epigenetics, and gut bacteria affect IBS, researchers aim to better understand its causes. This could lead to new tests and treatments that work well for individuals with IBS, offering hope for better managing their symptoms.

Mucosal immunology

Investigating mucosal immunology in individuals with IBS involves studying how the immune system responds and maintains the integrity of the mucosal barriers in the intestines. Researchers aim to develop therapies to strengthen the gut's defences against inflammation and other immune-related issues contributing to symptoms like bloating, diarrhoea, and constipation.

Advancements in mucosal immunology could lead to more targeted and personalised treatments for individuals with IBS in the future. By identifying specific immune responses and barriers unique to each patient, healthcare providers may be able to tailor therapies that address the underlying causes of their symptoms. This approach offers hope for improving the quality of life for individuals with IBS by reducing the frequency and severity of gastrointestinal symptoms they experience.

Microbiome-host interactions

Understanding how the genetics of the individual and the microbes in their gut interact to cause IBS can help develop targeted treatments. These treatments aim to balance the microbes in the gut and improve it's health.

This knowledge could pave the way for improved IBS treatments in the future. By focusing on the particular genetic and microbial factors underlying IBS, doctors might offer relief to individuals experiencing its symptoms, giving hope to those with IBS.

Longitudinal studies and clinical trials

Long-term studies and clinical trials are essential for advancing IBS treatment. Longitudinal studies follow people over time to understand how treatments work, and their safety. Testing new therapies in diverse groups helps identify effective treatments, allowing doctors to personalise care as needed. This offers hope to those with IBS by improving symptom relief and quality of life. It ensures treatments are thoroughly tested and safe before widespread use, giving individuals with IBS confidence in their effectiveness.

Conducting large-scale longitudinal studies and randomised controlled trials is essential to validate emerging therapies and interventions in diverse populations of individuals with IBS. This research ensures the efficacy and safety of new treatments.

Innovative treatment approaches

Future research aims to understand how changes in the gut microbiome relate to different diseases and how genes in both microbes and humans are affected. This could lead to better treatments for IBS and other conditions. As people age, they often experience oxidative stress and inflammation. While improving animal gut health has extended their lifespan, more human studies are needed. Prebiotics and dietary fibre can increase good bacteria in the gut, which would benefit overall well-being. However, some additives like propionate, used in food preservation, may cause insulin resistance.

Researchers understanding of gut bacteria has improved, and the findings suggested they also need to study other microbes like viruses and eukaryotes. For instance, bacteriophages (viruses that infect bacteria) and Blastocystis (a single-celled parasite) can affect gut health. Diet is crucial in influencing the gut microbiota and overall health. Instead of focusing on single nutrients, researchers now look at dietary patterns. A balanced diet helps keep your gut bacteria healthy, which can improve chronic conditions like diabetes, obesity, IBS, IBD, and depression.

One important research question is defining a healthy gut microbiome and how individuals can achieve it. Different people have different gut bacteria, explaining why some diets work better for others. New methods are needed to study these bacteria and their effects on health. Personalised medicine and nutrition, tailored to an individual's gut microbiome, could be the future of treatment. Researchers can create personalised interventions to improve gut health by understanding how diet and gut bacteria interact. Researchers are also exploring innovative microbiome treatments to manage conditions like IBS and IBD. Scientists aim to develop targeted therapies that reduce symptoms and enhance the quality of life for individuals with IBS by unravelling the impact of the gut microbiome on these conditions.

Community health implications

Understanding how gut bacteria affect community health is essential. Researchers are studying how different gut microbes help prevent diseases and maintain good health. This knowledge can lead to public health strategies that reduce gastrointestinal disorders worldwide.

Everyone's gut microbiome is unique and changes with age, diet, genetics, and medication. The research says using specially engineered bacteria is one advanced way to improve microbiome health. Unlike regular probiotics, these bacteria are designed to perform specific functions that can help regulate gut health. Using tools from synthetic biology, scientists can reprogram these bacteria to target particular diseases.

For example, these engineered bacteria could help with metabolic diseases, prevent cancer, and fight harmful pathogens. They produce substances like short-chain fatty acids (SCFAs) by fermenting dietary fibres, which have anti-inflammatory effects and improve gut health. SCFAs like butyrate can regulate appetite, reduce insulin resistance, and also promote fat burning.

Most of these treatments are still being tested but hold great promise. By closing the knowledge gaps about how microbes interact with each other and the human body, scientists hope to create better tools and treatments. This can offer new hope for individuals with IBS, reducing symptoms like wind, bloating, diarrhoea, and irregular bowel movements. Future therapies could lead to personalised treatments, helping people with IBS live healthier and happier lives.

Implications for public health

Understanding how different types of bacteria in the gut can affect health is vital to transforming personalised medicine and public health strategies. By promoting a healthy gut through specific diets and therapies that target the microbiome, researchers and scientists can lessen the impact of long-term digestive problems.

Ongoing efforts in medical research to explore microbiome diversity highlighted its potential to significantly improve health outcomes and advance personalised medicine. This research could lead the way in microbiome science and treatment for IBS, aiming to translate scientific advancements into practical clinical strategies that better manage and enhance outcomes for individuals with IBS. The research approach involved using the Blueprint persona method with a focus group of experts from various fields to identify the need for a mobile health (mHealth) intervention. This intervention promotes healthy lifestyles through nutrition, physical activity, meditation, and psychological support.

The study highlighted the need for further research to understand how mHealth services can help individuals with IBS manage their condition and enhance their quality of life. Integrating mHealth data with Electronic Health Records (EHR) and other professional data will provide vital insights to improve diagnosis and treatment.

It is crucial to study the feasibility, usability, and adaptability of personalised care plans that meet the diverse needs of those with IBS and conduct cost-effectiveness studies. This research will demonstrate how mHealth interventions impact IBS individuals' health outcomes and quality of life and potentially reduce healthcare costs over time.

Autoimmunity and IBS

Studies suggest there might be a link between gut bacteria and autoimmune conditions such as Rheumatoid arthritis, multiple sclerosis, and type 1 diabetes to name a few. In the study, some individuals with IBS showed signs of a slight immune response in their gut. Scientists are researching how gut bacteria interactions influence this response, aiming to understand the precise mechanisms involved. While IBS itself is not considered an autoimmune disease, some individuals with IBS display features similar to autoimmune diseases. They may also have a higher likelihood of developing autoimmune conditions. Scientists are actively studying how gut bacteria relate to various gut issues, including IBS. Further research is needed to fully understand the connections between gut bacteria, autoimmune responses, and IBS.

IBS treatments for adults and children

There is yet no cure for IBS, but the following treatments can help manage symptoms:
- **Ayurvedic treatments** for digestive health include therapies like Panchakarma, Shirodhara, Abhyanga, Basti (medicated enema), herbal remedies, as well as simple remedies like ginger tea, fennel seeds (saunf), buttermilk, and cumin water (jeera) for children. These treatments are tailored to meet individual needs, ensuring safe and effective management of digestive issues such as IBS. Panchakarma is an elaborate detoxification and rejuvenation treatment in Ayurveda that involves several stages aimed at cleansing the body and restoring dosha balance. It includes therapies like herbal massages, medicated enemas, and dietary adjustments tailored to individual needs. Shirodhara (oil pouring therapy), Abhyanga (oil massage), specific herbal remedies, and nutritional regulations focus on different aspects of health and wellness, including digestion. These treatments can complement Panchakarma but are more targeted and may be used individually depending on the person's specific health concerns and symptoms. Opt for an Ayurvedic practitioner or doctor who provides holistic health care based on individual constitution and balance of doshas.
- **Cognitive behavioural therapy (CBT)** helps those with IBS by focusing on how thoughts and behaviours influence IBS symptoms. It involves learning practical skills to manage stress and anxiety, which can aggravate IBS. CBT sessions are typically conducted with a therapist over time. It is recommended to consider CBT if IBS symptoms are significantly affecting daily life or if stress and anxiety are making symptoms worse. By addressing negative thinking patterns and behaviours, CBT aims to enhance the quality of life and reduce the impact of IBS symptoms. CBT is mainly for adults, but it can be adapted for children with the help of a professional.
- **Expressive writing** involves freely writing about thoughts and feelings connected to IBS symptoms. It is a private activity that can be done regularly, focusing on emotions and personal experiences. This method is beneficial when IBS symptoms are emotionally challenging or disrupt daily life. Expressive writing suits adults and older children who can write about their thoughts and feelings. Expressive writing helps individuals process and release emotions tied to IBS, potentially reducing stress and improving mental well-being. It is a valuable self-care practice distinct from journaling, typically documenting daily events and reflections. Instead, expressive writing explores and expresses emotions linked to managing symptoms of IBS. It focuses on understanding how these symptoms impact daily life and emotional well-being. Writing regularly can uncover triggers and patterns, offering a therapeutic approach to handling emotional challenges and enhancing overall wellness. This practice helps individuals gain insights into their condition, potentially leading to better symptom management and improved quality of life.
- **Gut-directed hypnotherapy** is where a therapist helps someone with IBS enter a relaxed or focused state using hypnosis. Gut-directed hypnotherapy is primarily used for adults, but it can be beneficial for children if done by a therapist experienced in paediatric hypnotherapy. This mindfulness-based stress reduction and cognitive-behavioural therapy has shown promising results in improving gut-brain interactions and easing symptoms. By addressing both the physical and emotional aspects of IBS, these techniques aim to provide comprehensive management. They are

helpful for individuals seeking to manage their condition effectively, potentially reducing symptoms and improving overall well-being.

Vagus nerve stimulation uses electrical impulses to enhance communication between the brain and gut by targeting the vagus nerve. While effective in different conditions, more research is needed to determine its specific use in IBS treatment. On the other hand, gut-directed hypnotherapy is preferred for its noninvasive method and potential psychological advantages in reducing IBS symptoms. The decision between these treatments depends on the individual patient's needs and response to therapy.

- **Coping mechanisms for children with IBS:** teaching your child how to cope with IBS involves showing them healthy ways to manage stress, such as through exercise, relaxation techniques, or talking to a trusted adult. Creating a supportive and caring home environment is essential. Teach children enjoyably and interactively, focusing on activities that bring them joy and help reduce their stress. Avoid unnecessary stressors and create a positive atmosphere at home. If your child struggles to handle stress alone, consider seeking help from a therapist. They can provide support in developing coping strategies and managing stress effectively. Supporting children with IBS means teaching them these skills and ensuring they feel supported and cared for at home.

- **The emerging market of microbiome-based products** covers a range of items that promote gut health and overall well-being. Examples include probiotics, live bacteria and yeasts that aid digestion, and prebiotics, fibres that nourish good gut bacteria. There are also postbiotics and metabolic byproducts of probiotics with health benefits. Moreover, microbiome testing kits analyse gut bacteria and offer personalised nutrition plans based on the results. These products balance gut microbiota, potentially enhancing digestive health and overall wellness. The emerging market of microbiome-based products is generally aimed at adults. However, some, like specific probiotics, can be suitable for children when supervised by a doctor. With increasing demand, it is vital to overcome regulatory and intellectual property challenges to ensure these products meet standards and are legally protected. This helps advance microbiome research and innovation, potentially enhancing treatments for conditions like IBS. It also improves safe healthcare practices and builds trust among consumers and healthcare providers, promoting long-term health benefits despite the absence of historical success data in microbiome-based products.

Individuals with IBS should consult their qualified healthcare professionals for personalised medical advice before seeking information about their specific diagnosis, treatment, or management of a condition or disorder.

CHAPTER RECAP:

Recent studies highlight the transformative potential of microbiome diversity in medical research, particularly in enhancing health outcomes and advancing personalised medicine. The role of the gut microbiome in influencing IBS symptoms is a significant focus of current research. Variations in gut bacteria composition may contribute to individual differences in symptom presentation and treatment response. Understanding these microbial dynamics could lead to innovative interventions like personalised probiotic therapies or microbiome-targeted dietary modifications tailored to each person's unique gut ecosystem. This promising research holds the potential to revolutionise IBS management in the future.

If dietary adjustments and medications do not reduce IBS symptoms, consulting with qualified healthcare professionals or an Ayurvedic practitioner may suggest exploring Panchakarma Ayurvedic treatment, gut-directed hypnotherapy, or cognitive behavioural therapy as potential beneficial treatments that promote long-term gut health. Treatment approaches for IBS range from dietary modifications and lifestyle changes to pharmacological interventions, with emerging therapies like gut-directed hypnotherapy showing promise. These therapies address various aspects, such as visceral hypersensitivity, alterations in gut neurotransmitters, and sensory processing. Moreover, methods like faecal microbiota transplantation and neuromodulation techniques are being explored.

Psychological factors play a significant role in IBS symptomatology. Techniques such as gut-directed hypnotherapy, mindfulness-based stress reduction, and cognitive-behavioural therapy have shown effectiveness in improving symptoms and quality of life for those with IBS. This emphasises the need for integrated care that combines diet and nutrition management with medical and behavioural treatments.

Future directions in IBS research highlight the need to focus on the role of microbiome dysbiosis and the potential for personalised treatment approaches based on individual microbiome profiles. Understanding individual variations in symptom presentation and response to treatment is essential for personalised management and improving individuals' overall quality of life. By embracing a comprehensive, microbiome-focused approach, individuals with IBS can reclaim their gut health and thrive beyond the limitations of their condition.

To further your understanding, explore additional resources, connect with supportive communities, and access the tools and guidance needed for lasting relief and optimal digestive well-being. **Remember**, every journey is unique, so be patient, stay proactive, and trust in your body's ability to heal and adapt. This balanced treatment and symptom management approach acknowledges the individuality of symptoms and the need for personalised solutions, offering hope for a deeper understanding and better future gut health.

Final Thoughts

"The well bred contradict other people. The wise contradict themselves." — Oscar Wilde

28. Empowering Readers to Take Control of Their Gut Health

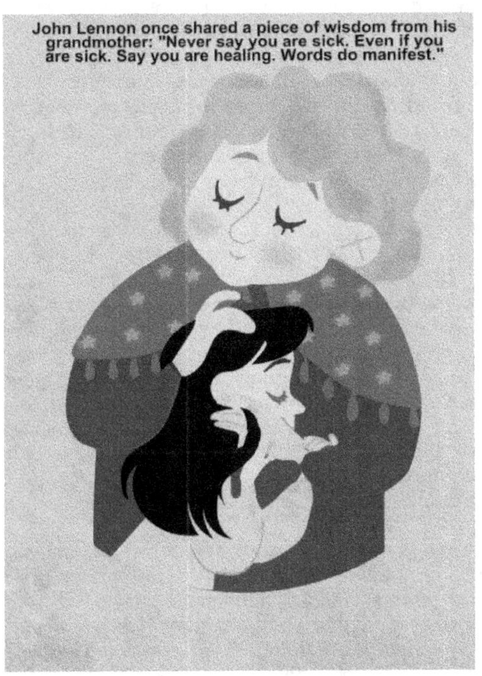

Original image by Ninikvaratskhelia. Edited by Jan Nallathamby

This book offers a comprehensive approach to gut health, drawing from personal experiences and coping strategies developed over 25 years with IBS-C. It highlights the importance of positive thinking and healthy habits in managing IBS symptoms, which affect all areas of life. Understanding food origins and embracing a holistic lifestyle enhances well-being. Mindful eating, small changes, and persistent effort are crucial for effective IBS symptom management.

Understanding how to effectively manage different IBS sub-types and body dosha types through portion control and balanced diets is essential for coping with IBS symptoms. Establishing realistic expectations, maintaining dietary variety, and employing effective coping strategies are necessary for long-term gut health and overall well-being. Avoiding food addictions like coffee and alcohol, which often trigger IBS symptoms, and prioritising diverse nutrient-rich superfoods such as millet, amla, and moringa are critical for maintaining optimal gut health. Embracing dietary diversity by cultivating a preference for a variety of nutrient-rich global foods, rather than simply indulging in flavourful options, is especially important for individuals managing IBS and nurturing a diverse gut microbiota.

Good nutrition includes integrating fermented foods like Indian dosa, Japanese natto, and sauerkraut into your daily diet, promoting beneficial gut bacteria. Ensuring adequate fibre intake from sources like powdered flax seeds and cluster beans reduces constipation. Fibre is essential for gut health as it supports digestion and maintains a balanced gut bacteria environment.

Imbalances in the gut microbiome, termed microbiome dysbiosis, can disturb the gut equilibrium, affecting digestion, immune function, and mental health and aggravating IBS symptoms. Healthy gut bacteria are vital for overall well-being, highlighting the importance of maintaining this balance. Restoring equilibrium through dietary adjustments, intermittent fasting, and probiotics is essential for optimising your gut ecosystem.

Managing weight is essential for staying healthy and preventing diseases. Tracking your Body Mass Index and using digital scales to measure body fat can help you monitor your progress accurately. Effective weight management helps control symptoms of conditions like IBS. It improves metabolic efficiency, lowering the likelihood of developing chronic illnesses like diabetes, heart disease, and certain cancers.

Using your hand to gauge food portions and employing apps to scrutinise ingredient labels are effective strategies for managing weight and improving digestive health. Monitoring your daily nutrition intake is pivotal in this regard. When managing IBS symptoms like bloating, it is important to check ingredients for hidden sugars or salts. Even minimal quantities spread over a few days can increase discomfort. It is sensible to skip ingredients that need to be clarified or are tricky to pronounce. Instead, focus on eating more natural foods.

Planning meals and steering clear of potential triggers such as gluten and, for some, onion and garlic are vital. Timing meals appropriately, ideally finishing your last meal before sunset, is also crucial. Opting for straightforward, fresh dishes with mild flavours helps reduce abdominal discomfort. It minimises mealtime anxiety, leading to improved digestive well-being. Your diet is more than just food; it is what you read, the people you spend time with, and what you hear and see. It is what you consume emotionally, spiritually and physically.

Understanding your life's purpose by exploring your Ikigai and engaging in personality type and dosha assessments can guide seeking support from loved ones, boosting emotional well-being, and positively influencing gut health. A supportive environment includes educating others about your IBS condition through proactive communication, setting healthy boundaries, and ensuring transparent, compelling dialogue. This approach promotes understanding and empathy, which are crucial for effectively managing IBS in social and work environments. A supportive approach significantly enhances an individual's ability to manage their symptoms of IBS effectively.

Forming a habit usually takes between three weeks to two months, depending on its complexity and how motivated you are. Health, nutrition, an active lifestyle, and positive thinking are vital for a fulfilling life. Establishing routines strengthens this foundation and aids in developing healthy habits over time.

Incorporating gentle movements throughout the day, which benefit your gut, alongside regular activities such as walking or Japanese Radio Taiso stretching exercises, promotes overall health. Tailoring dietary and lifestyle changes to fit individual needs and Ayurvedic principles supports holistic gut health management. Embracing mindfulness, intentional outdoor activities in nature, and self-care empowers individuals to discover personalised solutions for their well-being and daily life.

Getting enough consistent deep sleep and reviewing daily nutrient intake before bedtime is essential for health. Aligning with your body's natural biological cycles supports gut health. Establishing regular morning and night routines promotes stability and resilience in managing the unpredictable challenges associated with IBS.

Reducing excessive stress and preventing burnout involves planning your ideal week ahead and prioritising long-term health goals over immediate gains. This approach is crucial for mental resilience and gut health. Techniques like diaphragmatic breathing and expressive writing can effectively reduce stress levels. Maintaining a healthy stress balance is vital for gut health and sustainable symptom management.

Understanding your energy peaks helps prioritise activities that bring satisfaction and minimise stress. Effectively managing fatigue involves balancing workload, prioritising long-term goals, and ensuring adequate Vitamin D intake for overall well-being and professional success.

Successfully managing IBS over the long term involves continuously adapting to new information and advancements in gut microbiome research. Collaborating with healthcare professionals ensures personalised treatment plans tailored to individual needs.

Natural home remedies offer practical support for managing IBS flare-ups. Looking ahead, advancements in microbiome research show promising developments in IBS treatments. Long-term management involves thorough body tests to identify nutritional deficiencies, ongoing education, adapting to personal needs, and collaborating with healthcare professionals for tailored treatments. This approach nurtures a sense of curiosity and continuous learning.

Managing IBS effectively necessitates acknowledging that symptom management can fluctuate, and improvement may require time, patience, and ongoing effort.

Throughout life's journey, challenges arise that you can navigate with grace,
I believe in your strength and perseverance; you will find your rightful place.
When chronic pain and IBS symptoms cloud your path,
Tap into your inner strength, and let positivity last.
Believe in yourself, for strength resides within,
Stay active, and let the healing continue.

Wishing you good health and peace on your journey.

The information provided in this book is for educational purposes only and should not substitute professional medical advice. It is advisable to consult a qualified healthcare provider for personalised diagnosis and guidance specific to individual IBS health needs and conditions.

Additional Resources

Affiliate products:

Books:
- Chapter 21, **page 96**:
  - ✓ Time vs energy management: for more insights on building habits, consider reading 'Atomic Habits.' by James Clear: https://amzn.to/4cag7DU
- Chapter 23, **page 102**:
  - ✓ Further resources to help manage work stress consider reading 'The Body Keeps the Score: Mind, Brain, and Body in the Transformation of Trauma.' by Bessel van der Kolk: https://amzn.to/4cuBMqG
  - ✓ If childhood stress affects your IBS, check out 'The Deepest Well: Healing the Long-Term Effects of Childhood Adversity.' by Dr Nadine Burke Harris: https://amzn.to/3KAzI4g

Other products:
- Chapter 18:
  - ✓ **Page 66.** Microgreens: Explore a variety of vegetable and herb easy-to-grow home micro green sprouts with the 'Verdant Republic Microgreens Salad Seeds Mix | Fawn Collection- 5 Seeds Mix Packs | High Germination & Easy to Sprout | Over 16 Vegetable & Herbs Varieties incl Broccoli, Radish, Kale': https://amzn.to/3yzefWH
  - ✓ **Page 70.** Nourishing nut options: 'Sunburst Snacks Crispy and Spicy Wasabi Coated Peas, Resealable and Recyclable Packaging, 1KG': https://amzn.to/3V5Nqki
  - ✓ **Page 79.** Honey choices for IBS: 'Forest Field Honey' from the Baltic Honey Shop Store': https://amzn.to/3vXQbM0
  - ✓ **Page 80.** Baking with gluten-dairy-wheat-nut free ingredients: use the discount code JANN20 to get 20% off everything with global shipping to around 18 countries: https://creativenaturesuperfoods.co.uk/recipe_category/meal-type/
- Chapter 20, **page 90**:
  - ✓ Using a digital smart scale can help manage IBS through calorie and fat monitoring. 'Bluetooth Body Fat Scales, INSMART Smart Digital Bathroom Weight Weighing Scales for Body Composition Analyser with Smart APP, Body Composition Fitbit Scales for Fitness,': https://amzn.to/3R4oTL9
- Chapter 25, **page 108**:
  - ✓ Experience relief from constipation with the natural benefits of fresh coconut water, available at https://amzn.to/3UsjWhq

Weblinks cited in this book for your quick access:

- Chapter 3, **page 16**: Potential Impact of Body Types on IBS:
  - ✓ The 10-minute free survey Dosha quiz to assess your body Ayurvedic type and get free tips via email to help with IBS symptom management: https://www.banyanbotanicals.com/info/dosha-quiz/
- Chapter 16, **Pages 59-60**: Incorporate food and symptoms tracking into meal planning:
  - ✓ IBS Tracker, Food Diary, Allergy, Medicine and Supplement Tracking Sheet, Diet Tracker, Meal Planner, Daily Health Planner, Symptom Tracker by Etsy seller FRGLMAMA: https://www.etsy.com/uk/listing/1074201132/ibs-tracker-food-diary-allergy-medicine?ga_order=highest_reviews&ga_search_type=all&ga_view_type=gallery&ga_search_query=ibs&ref=sr_gallery-1-16&pro=1&sts=1&dd=1&content_source=f47fde962dc9825699d53239a6dac74e1a3
  - ✓ FODMAP Diet Food Guide, Low and High FODMAP Grocery List, IBS Food List, Food Chart, Nutrition Dietitian Worksheet (Digital Printable) by Etsy seller LearningHealthCo: https://www.etsy.com/uk/listing/1449671967/fodmap-diet-food-guide-low-and-high?ga_order=highest_reviews&ga_search_type=all&ga_view_type=gallery&ga_search_qu

ery=high+food+map&ref=sr_gallery-1-
2&dd=1&content_source=5b24ee28e5418c6236c510e41ee0202d9461da51%2
- ✓ IBS Diet, Irritable Bowel Syndrome, Food List, Grocery List, Food Guide, What To Eat, What Not To Eat, Gut Health Nutrition, PDF Download by Etsy seller TheSecretPrintables: https://www.etsy.com/uk/listing/1647695835/ibs-diet-irritable-bowel-syndrome-food?ga_order=most_relevant&ga_search_type=all&ga_view_type=gallery&ga_search_query=ibs&ref=sr_gallery-1-
47&dd=1&content_source=e991a4d2303561efc4b243089d70634fc4cc0f73%253A16476
- ✓ Complete FODMAP shopping list - Low FODMAP and high FODMAP food list - FODMAP diet grocery list – FODMAP chart for irritable bowel syndrome by Etsy seller NutriWellness: https://www.etsy.com/uk/listing/1525065388/complete-fodmap-shopping-list-low-fodmap?ga_order=highest_reviews&ga_search_type=all&ga_view_type=gallery&ga_search_query=high+food+map&ref=sr_gallery-1-
16&pro=1&sts=1&dd=1&content_source=4069a518669da8cae1cbe039
- ✓ FODMAP IBS Food List and Low FODMAP Treats, Food Chart Nutrition Guide for IBS Meal Plan and Gut Health, Gluten-Free Diet Meal Prep Grocery by Etsy seller TheMichellicious: https://www.etsy.com/uk/listing/1671849592/fodmap-ibs-food-list-and-low-fodmap?ga_order=most_relevant&ga_search_type=all&ga_view_type=gallery&ga_search_query=ibs&ref=sr_gallery-1-
11&pro=1&pop=1&dd=1&content_source=ef2a22d644f76b3efe687993db73f753f30dd0ca%

- Chapter 17, **page 62**:
  - ✓ Morning routine habit 3: write a 5- minute daily journal with a stress log:
    - o Tummy Trouble Tracker by Etsy seller StardustStickers: https://www.etsy.com/uk/listing/580994988/tummy-trouble-tracker?ga_order=highest_reviews&ga_search_type=all&ga_view_type=gallery&ga_search_query=ibs+tracker+sticker&ref=sr_gallery-1-
12&content_source=72b1f2a74b0dfa7060c382c40dab77ce0b189761%253A580994988 &
    - o 35 Cute Happy Gut/IBS Planner Stickers by Etsy seller HappyCutieStudio: https://www.etsy.com/uk/listing/540986664/35-cute-happy-gutibs-planner-stickers?ga_order=highest_reviews&ga_search_type=all&ga_view_type=gallery&ga_search_query=ibs+tracker+sticker&ref=sc_gallery-1-
2&local_signal_search=1&search_preloaded_img=1&plkey=3da4
  - ✓ Morning routine habit 5: stretching exercises for 7 minutes followed by 2 minutes weights and 5 minutes yoga:
    - o Japanese Radio Taiso exercise routine: ラジオ体操 第一 第二 首 by album-chat: https://www.youtube.com/watch?v=RBnsvftHQtU
    - o Malasana walk yoga for women! #yogateacher #yogawithkamya #onlineyogaclass #shortsvideo #yogaforweightloss #fyp: https://youtube.com/shorts/cQAbfWiRi2o?si=Q13Y3yUCi_QSFuMx
- Chapter 21, **page 93**: Assessing your career fit and well-being:
  - ✓ Free personality test to figure out if your job is right for you and if it makes you happy, which impacts IBS symptom management at psality.com/test-en/

Recommended books on IBS:

- Take Control of Your IBS: The Complete Guide to Managing Your Symptoms by Peter J. Whorwell, 2017.
- Man Food by Ian Marber, 2019.

Other groups and networks:

- The IBS network: www.ibsnetwork.org
- Self Help IBS Group: www.ibsgroup.org
- Steps for Stress: www.stepsforstress.org

Renowned international IBS organisations:

- American Gastroenterological Association (AGA)
- Asian Neurogastroenterology and Motility Association (ANMA)
- British Society of Gastroenterology (BSG)
- Canadian Society of Intestinal Research (CSIR)
- European Society for Neurogastroenterology and Motility (ESNM)
- Gastroenterological Society of Australia (GESA)
- International Foundation for Functional Gastrointestinal Disorders (IFFGD)
- International Foundation for Gastrointestinal Disorders (IFFGD)
- Irritable Bowel Syndrome Network (IBS Network, UK)
- Rome Foundation

References

Introduction

page 10. 'For example, a study in "Digestive Diseases and Sciences" in 2021 estimated that IBS affects about 10-15% of women...', Tai Zhang, Xiangxue Ma, Wende Tian, Jiaqi Zhang, Yuchen Wei, Beihua Zhang, Fengyun Wang and Xudong Tang, 'Global Research Trends in Irritable Bowel Syndrome: A Bibliometric and Visualized Study', 27 June 2022, https://www.ncbi.nlm.nih.gov/pmc/articles/PMC9271748/

page 10. 'According to the National Institute of Diabetes and Digestive and Kidney Diseases (NIDDK), women are more prone to symptoms...', NIDDK, 'Definition & Facts for Irritable Bowel Syndrome', November 2017, https://www.niddk.nih.gov/health-information/digestive.

page 10. 'Iron supplements may cause constipation in pregnant women...', Zoe Tolkien, Lynne Stecher, Adrian P Mander, Dora I A Pereira and Jonathan J Powell, 'Ferrous Sulfate Supplementation Causes Significant Gastrointestinal Side-Effects in Adults: A Systematic Review and Meta-Analysis', 20 February 2015, https://www.ncbi.nlm.nih.gov/pmc/articles/PMC4336293/

page 10. 'Each subtype of IBS comes with it's symptoms and management challenges...', Kexin Wang, Huan Liu, Jingjing Liu, Liyuan Han, Zheng Kang, Libo Liang, Shengchao Jiang, Nan Meng, Peiwen Chen, Qiao Xu, Qunhong Wu and Yanhua Hao, 'Factors related to irritable bowel syndrome and differences among subtypes: A cross-sectional study in the UK Biobank', 26 August 2022, https://www.ncbi.nlm.nih.gov/pmc/articles/PMC9458926/

page 10. Different types of IBS Stacy Menees and William Chey, 'The gut microbiome and irritable bowel syndrome', 9 July 2018, https://www.ncbi.nlm.nih.gov/pmc/articles/PMC6039952/

page 13. Rumi. "Maybe you are searching among the branches, for what only appears in the roots." TheGoldenQuotes.net, https://www.thegoldenquotes.net/best-100-public-domain-quotes-of-all-time-collection-01/best-100-public-domain-quotes-of-all-time-collection-04

Chapter 1

page 13. Fyodor Dostoevsky. "Be the sun and all will see you." TheGoldenQuotes.net, https://www.thegoldenquotes.net/best-100-public-domain-quotes-of-all-time-collection-01/best-100-public-domain-quotes-of-all-time-collection-04

page 13. 'The diagnosis of IBS-C is primarily symptom-based and follows established guidelines such as the Rome IV criteria, the latest version published in 2016...,' Brian E Lacy and Nihal K Patel, 'Rome Criteria and a Diagnostic Approach to Irritable Bowel Syndrome', 26 October 2017, https://www.mdpi.com/2077-0383/6/11/99

Chapter 2

page 15. Christiaan Huygens. "I do not believe anything very certainly, but everything very probably." TheGoldenQuotes.net, https://www.thegoldenquotes.net/best-100-public-domain-quotes-of-all-time-collection-01/best-100-public-domain-quotes-of-all-time-collection-03

Chapter 3

page 16. Lewis Carroll. "I can't go back to yesterday, because I was a different person then." TheGoldenQuotes.net, https://www.thegoldenquotes.net/best-100-public-domain-quotes-of-all-time-collection-01/best-100-public-domain-quotes-of-all-time-collection-03

page 16. Banyan Botanicals, 'Dosha Quiz', https://www.banyanbotanicals.com/pages/dosha

page 16. 'The Vata dosha is associated with elements of air and ether…', Unnikrishnan Payyappallimana and Padma Venkatasubramanian, 'Exploring Ayurvedic Knowledge on Food and Health for Providing Innovative Solutions to Contemporary Healthcare', 31 March 2016, https://www.ncbi.nlm.nih.gov/pmc/articles/PMC4815005/

page 17. 'Dr. Sharda Ayurveda, India's leading Ayurvedic clinic, focuses on balancing the doshas with…', Dr Sharda Ayurveda, 'The natural way to heal Irritable Bowel Syndrome-C via Ayurveda', 22 May 2024, https://drshardaayurveda.com/blogs/digestive

Chapter 4

page 19. Vladimir Lenin. "You must have your heart on fire and your brain on ice." TheGoldenQuotes.net, https://www.thegoldenquotes.net/best-100-public-domain-quotes-of-all-time-collection-01/best-100-public-domain-quotes-of-all-time-collection-02

page 19. Democritus. "It is hard to fight desire; but to control it is the sign of a reasonable man." TheGoldenQuotes.net, https://www.thegoldenquotes.net/best-100-public-domain-quotes-of-all-time-collection-01/best-100-public-domain-quotes-of-all-time-collection-02

Chapter 5

page 20. Louisa May Alcott. "It's amazing how lovely common things become, if one only knows how to look at them." TheGoldenQuotes.net, https://www.thegoldenquotes.net/best-100-public-domain-quotes-of-all-time-collection-01/best-100-public-domain-quotes-of-all-time-collection-02

Chapter 6

page 21. Francois Rabelais. "A child is not a vase to be filled, but a fire to be lit." TheGoldenQuotes.net, https://www.thegoldenquotes.net/best-100-public-domain-quotes-of-all-time-collection-01/best-100-public-domain-quotes-of-all-time-collection-02

Chapter 7

page 23. Jane Austen. "The less said the better." TheGoldenQuotes.net, https://www.thegoldenquotes.net/best-100-public-domain-quotes-of-all-time-collection-01/best-100-public-domain-quotes-of-all-time-collection-03

page 24. 'research suggests that it is not necessary to have a bowel movement every day. The frequency of bowel movements can vary from person to person, and it is considered normal to have anywhere from three bowel movements per week to three per…', Johannes PJohnson-Martínez, Christian Diener, Anne E Levine, Tomasz Wilmanski, David L Suskind, Alexandra Ralevski, Jennifer Hadlock, Andrew T Magis, Leroy Hood, Noa Rappaport and Sean M Gibbons, 'Generally-healthy individuals with aberrant bowel movement frequencies show enrichment for microbially-derived blood metabolites associated with reduced kidney function', 6 March 2023, https://www.ncbi.nlm.nih.gov/pmc/articles/PMC10028848/

page 25. 'Bristol stool chart' Image courtesy of Cabot Health. Wikimedia Commons, https://commons.wikimedia.org/wiki/File:Bristol_stool_chart.svg. Used under Creative commons license.

page 27. Margaret Fuller. "If you have the knowledge, let others light their candles in it." TheGoldenQuotes.net, https://www.thegoldenquotes.net/best-100-public-domain-quotes-of-all-time-collection-01/best-100-public-domain-quotes-of-all-time-collection-02

Chapter 8

page 27. John Keates. "Nothing ever becomes real till experienced." TheGoldenQuotes.net, https://www.thegoldenquotes.net/best-100-public-domain-quotes-of-all-time-collection-01/best-100-public-domain-quotes-of-all-time-collection-02

Chapter 9

page 29. Theodore N. Vail. "Real difficulties can be overcome, it is only the imaginary ones that are unconquerable." TheGoldenQuotes.net, https://www.thegoldenquotes.net/best-100-public-domain-quotes-of-all-time-collection-01/best-100-public-domain-quotes-of-all-time-collection-04

Chapter 10

page 30. Hafez. "Never give up. No one knows what's going to happen next." TheGoldenQuotes.net, https://www.thegoldenquotes.net/best-100-public-domain-quotes-of-all-time-collection-01/best-100-public-domain-quotes-of-all-time-collection-02

Chapter 11

page 31. Plato. "The beginning is the most important part of the work." TheGoldenQuotes.net, https://www.thegoldenquotes.net/best-100-public-domain-quotes-of-all-time-collection-01

page 31. 'Research indicates that inadequate levels of Vitamin D might contribute to both IBS and mental health conditions, and it is also believed to influence central hypersensitivity. However, chronic…', Mental health and malabsorption Mohamed Abuelazm, Shoaib Muhammad, Mohamed Gamal, Fatma Labieb, Mostafa Atef Amin, Basel Abdelazeem, and James Robert Brašić, 'The Effect of Vitamin D Supplementation on the Severity of Symptoms and the Quality of Life in Irritable Bowel Syndrome Patients: A Systematic Review and Meta-Analysis of Randomized Controlled Trials', 24 June 2022, https://www.ncbi.nlm.nih.gov/pmc/articles/PMC9268238/

Chapter 12

page 33. 'Nathaniel Hawthorne. "Times flies over us, but leaves its shadow behind." TheGoldenQuotes.net, https://www.thegoldenquotes.net/best-100-public-domain-quotes-of-all-time-collection-01/best-100-public-domain-quotes-of-all-time-collection-04

page 34. 'black chickpeas are often a better choice for those with IBS because they have increased fibre content and a reduced glycemic index compared to white chickpeas…', Fit Tuber, '5 Things to Instantly Make Your Atta a Superfood (#2 will Surprise you)', 31 May 2024, see https://www.youtube.com/watch?v=VQfHP5Injhg

Chapter 13

page 35. Johann Wolfgang von Goethe. "If you want to make life easy, make it hard." TheGoldenQuotes.net, https://www.thegoldenquotes.net/best-100-public-domain-quotes-of-all-time-collection-01

page 35. Abraham Lincoln. "The best way to predict the future is to create it." TheGoldenQuotes.net, https://www.thegoldenquotes.net/best-100-public-domain-quotes-of-all-time-collection-01/best-100-public-domain-quotes-of-all-time-collection-03

page 35. 'Studies suggest that specific probiotic strains like Lactobacillus Plantarum and Bifidobacterium Breve could reduce IBS-C symptoms like bloating and abdominal…', Lakshmi Satish Kumar, Lakshmi

References

Sree Pugalenthi, Mahlika Ahmad, Sanjana Reddy, Zineb Barkhane and Jalal Elmadi, 'Probiotics in Irritable Bowel Syndrome: A Review of Their Therapeutic Role', 18 April 2022, https://www.ncbi.nlm.nih.gov/pmc/articles/PMC9116469/

page 36. 'There are two main types of fermentation aerobic and anaerobic. Aerobic fermentation needs...', Dr Pal, 'Celebrity Nutritionist Ryan Fernando Delves into Anti-Aging, Sugar Craving & Restaurant Food Concerns', 15 March 2024, see https://www.youtube.com/watch?v=un3--vdM4bE

page 37. 'The USDA tested baby foods, finding fewer pesticides in non-organic options than in whole fruits and vegetables, but still detected residues in 38% of products. Studies link pesticides to health...', Cheryl Callen, Jatinder Bhatia, Laura Czerkies, William J Klish and George M Gray, 'Challenges and Considerations When Balancing the Risks of Contaminants with the Benefits of Fruits and Vegetables for Infants and Toddlers', 24 October 2018, https://www.ncbi.nlm.nih.gov/pmc/articles/PMC6266946/

page 38. 'Selection of foods from diverse cultures that support a healthy gut microbiome' table. Natasha K Leeuwendaal, Catherine Stanton, Paul W O'Toole and Tom P Beresford, 'Fermented Foods, Health and the Gut Microbiome', 6 April 2022, https://www.ncbi.nlm.nih.gov/pmc/articles/PMC9003261/

Chapter 14

page 40. Mark Twain. "Good friends, good books, and a sleepy conscience: this is the ideal life." TheGoldenQuotes.net, https://www.thegoldenquotes.net/best-100-public-domain-quotes-of-all-time-collection-01/best-100-public-domain-quotes-of-all-time-collection-03

page 41. 'Research suggests that consuming carbohydrates, like whole grains, provides brain fuel, keeping your mind sharp and clear when glucose levels are consistent in each meal. Fill half your plate with vegetables...', and 'Image by British Heart Foundation 'How to get portion sizes right', British Heart Foundation, 'Food Portions', https://www.bhf.org.uk/informationsupport/support/healthy-living/healthy-eating. Written permission obtained.

page 42. 'Research suggests that late-night eating can disrupt circadian rhythms, our body's natural daily sleep-wake cycle clock...', Gregory D M Potter, Debra J Skene, Josephine Arendt, Janet E Cade, Peter J Grant and Laura J Hardie, 'Circadian Rhythm and Sleep Disruption: Causes, Metabolic Consequences, and Countermeasures', 20 October 2016, https://www.ncbi.nlm.nih.gov/pmc/articles/PMC5142605/

page 44. 'Adequate water intake softens stools, making them easier to pass, essential for those with IBS-C...', Asma Salari-Moghaddam, Ammar Hassanzadeh Keshteli, Ahmad Esmaillzadeh and Peyman Adibi, 'Water consumption and prevalence of irritable bowel syndrome among adults', 24 January 2020, https://www.ncbi.nlm.nih.gov/pmc/articles/PMC6980581/

page 46. 'Coconut oil is considered the best because it is safe to consume and has anti-inflammatory, antibacterial, and antimicrobial properties...', Julian Woolley, Tatjana Gibbons, Kajal Patel and Roberto Saccoc, 'The effect of oil pulling with coconut oil to improve dental hygiene and oral health: A systematic review', 27 August 2020, https://www.ncbi.nlm.nih.gov/pmc/articles/PMC7475120/

page 46. 'The research underscores the pivotal role of social support and engaging activities in enhancing mental and physical health, particularly in managing chronic conditions like IBS...', Mihaela Fadgyas Stanculete, Abdulrahman Ismaiel, Stefan-Lucian Popa and Octavia Oana Capatina, 'Irritable Bowel Syndrome and Resilience', 22 June 2023, https://www.ncbi.nlm.nih.gov/pmc/articles/PMC10342810/

page 47. 'Studies confirm footstools improve posture and reduce straining, particularly with IBS-C, leading to a more comfortable toilet experience...', Rohan M Modi, Alice Hinton, Daniel Pinkhas, Royce Groce, Marty M Meyer, Gokulakrishnan Balasubramanian, Edward Levine and Peter P Stanich, 'Implementation of a Defecation Posture Modification Device ', 11 February 2019, https://www.ncbi.nlm.nih.gov/pmc/articles/PMC6382038/

page 47. 'Neem is known for its anti-inflammatory and antibacterial properties...', Marina R Wylie and D Scott Merrell, 'The Antimicrobial Potential of the Neem Tree Azadirachta indica', 30 May 2022 https://www.ncbi.nlm.nih.gov/pmc/articles/PMC9195866/

page 48. 'The International Journal of Environmental Sciences & Natural Resources research focuses on "The Dirty Dozen Cleaning Products at Home." These include air...', Derrick A Balladin, 'The Dirty Dozen Cleaning Products at Home', 5 June 2020, https://www.researchgate.net/publication/348762787_The_Dirty_Dozen_Cleaning_Products_at_Home

Chapter 15

page 50. Leo Tolstoy. "Everyone thinks of changing the world, but no one thinks of changing himself." TheGoldenQuotes.net, https://www.thegoldenquotes.net/best-100-public-domain-quotes-of-all-time-collection-01/best-100-public-domain-quotes-of-all-time-collection-02

Chapter 16

page 56. Marcel Proust. "My destination is no longer a place, rather a new way of seeing." TheGoldenQuotes.net, https://www.thegoldenquotes.net/best-100-public-domain-quotes-of-all-time-collection-01/best-100-public-domain-quotes-of-all-time-collection-02

page 57. 'IBS treatment types' image content from NIDDK, 'Treatment for Irritable Bowel Syndrome How do doctors treat IBS?', November 2017, https://www.niddk.nih.gov/health-information/digestive-diseases/irritable-bowel-syndrome/treatment

page 59. Francis Scott Fitzgerald. "Experience is the name so many people give to their mistakes." TheGoldenQuotes.net, https://www.thegoldenquotes.net/best-100-public-domain-quotes-of-all-time-collection-01/best-100-public-domain-quotes-of-all-time-collection-02

Chapter 17

page 61. Victor Hugo. "Don't educate your children to be rich. Educate them to be happy, so they know the value of things, not the price." TheGoldenQuotes.net, https://www.thegoldenquotes.net/best-100-public-domain-quotes-of-all-time-collection-01/best-100-public-domain-quotes-of-all-time-collection-03

Chapter 18

page 65. Lord Chesterfield. "The less one has to do, the less time one finds to do it in." TheGoldenQuotes.net, https://www.thegoldenquotes.net/best-100-public-domain-quotes-of-all-time-collection-01/best-100-public-domain-quotes-of-all-time-collection-03

page 69. 'Including these top 9 nuts in your diet can be a valuable source of dietary fibre, which is beneficial for digestive health and managing IBS symptoms. Almonds...', Magdalena Woźniak, Agnieszka Waśkiewicz and Izabela Ratajczak, 'The Content of Phenolic Compounds and Mineral Elements in Edible Nuts', 6 July 2022, https://www.ncbi.nlm.nih.gov/pmc/articles/PMC9316459/

page 72. 'The collagen in chicken broth promotes the growth of beneficial bacteria in the gut, supporting an overall healthy...', Der-jen Hsu, Chia-wei Lee, Wei-choung Tsai and Yeh-chung Chien, 'Essential and toxic metals in animal bone broths',18 July 2017, https://www.ncbi.nlm.nih.gov/pmc/articles/PMC5533136/

page 73. 'Five excellent vegetarian sources of calcium include a pinch of edible limestone mixed in curd, sesame seeds...', Fit Tuber, '5 Foods that have More Calcium than Milk (Get Stronger Bones)', 28 June 2024, see https://www.youtube.com/watch?v=s5by_uGGkX0

page 73. 'Amaranth millet is 3.75 times more nutritious in calcium...', and 'Ragi has the highest calcium content of all millets...', Gayathri Balakrishnan and Renée Goodrich Schneider, 'The Role of Amaranth, Quinoa, and Millets for the Development of Healthy, Sustainable Food Products—A *Concise* Review', Table 3: Mineral content of ancient and common grains, 13 August 2022, https://www.ncbi.nlm.nih.gov/pmc/articles/PMC9407507/

page 76. 'White foods, notably "bad carbs" such as sugar and foods made from white flour, are often blamed for contributing to the obesity epidemic...', Yanni Papanikolaou, 'Pasta Consumption Is Linked to Greater Nutrient Intakes and Improved Diet Quality in American Children and Adults, and Beneficial Weight-Related Outcomes Only in Adult Females', 7 August 2020, https://www.ncbi.nlm.nih.gov/pmc/articles/PMC7426435/

page 79. 'Aim for less than 2000 mg/day of salt for adults, equivalent to less than 5 g/day, just under a teaspoon. For children aged 2–15 years...', Teresa Partearroyo, M de Lourdes Samaniego-Vaesken, Emma Ruiz, Javier Aranceta-Bartrina, Ángel Gil, Marcela González-Gross, Rosa M Ortega, Lluis Serra-Majem and Gregorio Varela-Moreiras, 'Sodium Intake from Foods Exceeds Recommended Limits in the Spanish Population: The ANIBES Study', 14 October 2019, https://www.ncbi.nlm.nih.gov/pmc/articles/PMC6835313/

page 82. 'Garlic and onions can make food tasty, but they contain fructans, which can mainly upset your stomach as it is not fully absorbed in the small intestine...', Dakota Rhys Jones, Chu K Yao and Peter R Gibson, 'Perceived food intolerances can guide personalization of the FODMAP diet but not the choice of dietary intervention', 28 November 2023, https://www.ncbi.nlm.nih.gov/pmc/articles/PMC10684989/

page 84. 'Self-created table by Jan Nallathamby content from PubMed Central on food combinations to avoid for IBS management...', Maleesha Jayasinghe, Vinuri Karunanayake, Ali Mohtashim, Dilushini Caldera, Piyalka Mendis, Omesh Prathiraja, Fatemeh Rashidi, and John A Damianos, 'The Role of Diet in the Management of Irritable Bowel Syndrome: A Comprehensive Review',15 February 2024, https://www.ncbi.nlm.nih.gov/pmc/articles/PMC10944297/

page 85. 'They are gentle on your stomach and can help you clear your bowels easier. If you are dealing with a runny poop, opt for bananas that...', Herlina Marta, Yana Cahyana, Mohamad Djali and Giffary Pramafisi, 'The Properties, Modification, and Application of Banana Starch', 29 July 2022, https://www.ncbi.nlm.nih.gov/pmc/articles/PMC9370678/

multiple pages across this chapter. Certain food and nutrition guidelines, suitable IBS foods, quantities and alternatives. Guy's & St Thomas' NHS Foundation Trust & King's College London, 'Suitable Products for the Low FODMAP Diet', 'Reintroducing FODMAPs and Long-Term Self Management' and 'Reducing Fermentable Carbohydrates the Low FODMAP Way'. January 2022 and October 2021 booklets. Written permission obtained.

Chapter 19

page 86. Thomas Carlyle. "He who has health, has hope; and he who has hope, has everything." TheGoldenQuotes.net, https://www.thegoldenquotes.net/best-100-public-domain-quotes-of-all-time-collection-01

page 87. 'Focus on getting deep sleep, about 20-25% of your total sleep, which is fundamental for physical and mental recovery...', Brett A Dolezal, Eric V Neufeld, David M Boland, Jennifer L Martin and Christopher B Cooper, 'Interrelationship between Sleep and Exercise: A Systematic Review', 26 March 2017, https://www.ncbi.nlm.nih.gov/pmc/articles/PMC5385214/

page 87. 'To improve sleep, manage stress, and support digestion, follow your natural body cycles. The liver detoxifies the body between 1 a.m. and 3 a.m...', Chinmayee Panda, Slavko Komarnytsky, Michelle Norton Fleming, Carissa Marsh, Keri Barron, Sara Le Brun-Blashka and Brandon Metzger, 'Guided

Metabolic Detoxification Program Supports Phase II Detoxification Enzymes and Antioxidant Balance in Healthy Participants', 6 May 2023, https://www.ncbi.nlm.nih.gov/pmc/articles/PMC10181083/

Chapter 20

page 89. Alexander Pope. "The only time you run out of chances is when you stop taking them." TheGoldenQuotes.net, https://www.thegoldenquotes.net/best-100-public-domain-quotes-of-all-time-collection-01/best-100-public-domain-quotes-of-all-time-collection-04

page 89. 'As we age, our cells' powerhouses, called mitochondria, may not work as well due to stress, inflammation, and genetics. While it is true…' Iñigo San-Millán, 'The Key Role of Mitochondrial Function in Health and Disease', 23 March 2023, https://www.ncbi.nlm.nih.gov/pmc/articles/PMC10135185/

page 90. 'Self-created table by Jan Nallathamby content from The Centers for Disease Control and Prevention 'How to Measure and Interpret Weight Status'. The Centers for Disease Control and Prevention, 'How to Measure and Interpret Weight Status', 3 June 2022, https://www.cdc.gov/healthyweight/assessing/index.html

page 91. 'Self-created table by Jan Nallathamby content from The Centers for Disease Control and Prevention 'Waist Circumference', The Centers for Disease Control and Prevention, 'Vital and Health Statistics', January 2019, https://www.cdc.gov/nchs/data/series/sr_02/sr02_182-508.pdf

page 92. 'For instance, a TDEE (Total Daily Energy Expenditure) calorie calculator can assist in determining your daily calorie requirements…', Andrew P Hills, Najat Mokhtar and Nuala M Byrne, 'Assessment of Physical Activity and Energy Expenditure: An Overview of Objective Measures', 16 June 2014, https://www.ncbi.nlm.nih.gov/pmc/articles/PMC4428382/

page 93. Mahatma Gandhi. "Earth provides enough to satisfy every man's needs, but not every man's greed." TheGoldenQuotes.net, https://www.thegoldenquotes.net/best-100-public-domain-quotes-of-all-time-collection-01/best-100-public-domain-quotes-of-all-time-collection-04

Chapter 21

page 93. Oscar Wilde. "All great ideas are dangerous." TheGoldenQuotes.net, https://www.thegoldenquotes.net/best-100-public-domain-quotes-of-all-time-collection-01/best-100-public-domain-quotes-of-all-time-collection-02

Chapter 22

page 96. Washington Irving. "Great minds have purpose, others have wishes." TheGoldenQuotes.net https://www.thegoldenquotes.net/best-100-public-domain-quotes-of-all-time-collection-01/best-100-public-domain-quotes-of-all-time-collection-03

page 96. 'Managing time involves eliminating distractions while managing energy means being mindful of when distractions affect us…', Rowena Tsai, 'the one productivity system you need: time vs energy management (ep. 1)', 15 August 2020, see https://www.youtube.com/watch?v=gDgk7rsy2lk

Chapter 23

page 99. John D. Rockefeller Jr. "The secret of success is to do the common thing uncommonly well." TheGoldenQuotes.net, https://www.thegoldenquotes.net/best-100-public-domain-quotes-of-all-time-collection-01/best-100-public-domain-quotes-of-all-time-collection-03

page 99. 'Stress affects both our minds and bodies, potentially resulting in serious health issues like heart disease, a weakened immune system, digestive problems, and chronic pain…', Yun-Zi Liu, Yun-Xia

References

Wang and Chun-Lei Jiang, 'Inflammation: The Common Pathway of Stress-Related Diseases', 20 June 2017, https://www.ncbi.nlm.nih.gov/pmc/articles/PMC5476783/

page 99. 'A well-rested mind operates more efficiently, producing sharper thinking and reduced errors. Studies show that these techniques can cut stress when practised consistently and with intention, which is impressive and can help with IBS symptoms to manage work-related stress...', Vijay Kumar Chattu, Md Dilshad Manzar, Soosanna Kumary, Deepa Burman, David Warren Spence and Seithikurippu R Pandi-Perumal, 'The Global Problem of Insufficient Sleep and Its Serious Public Health Implications', 20 December 2018, https://www.ncbi.nlm.nih.gov/pmc/articles/PMC6473877/

page 100. 'This aids in progressive muscle relaxation, which can reduce symptoms like stomach cramps, brain fog, or anxiety associated with IBS...', Larissa Hetterich and Andreas Stengel, 'Psychotherapeutic Interventions in Irritable Bowel Syndrome', 30 April 2020, https://www.ncbi.nlm.nih.gov/pmc/articles/PMC7205029/

page 100. "I get to do this" instead of "I have to do this...",Ali Abdaal, 'Shift your mindset', 20 June 2024, see https://youtube.com/shorts/zdR5t5wuRac?si=ERyHmfzKhvd0-06c

page 101. 'To ease work-related anxiety, use oils like lavender, which are known for their calming effects and for reducing stress...', Giselle A Borges e Soares, Tanima Bhattacharya, Tulika Chakrabarti, Priti Tagde and Simona Cavalu, 'Exploring Pharmacological Mechanisms of Essential Oils on the Central Nervous System', 22 December 2021, https://www.ncbi.nlm.nih.gov/pmc/articles/PMC8747111/

Chapter 24

page 103. Walt Whitman. "Either define the moment or the moment will define you." TheGoldenQuotes.net, https://www.thegoldenquotes.net/best-100-public-domain-quotes-of-all-time-collection-01

page 103. 'A survey from April to June 2022 collected data from 1,800 people aged 18-25. Most of the participants were females (53%) from...', Waleed M Alhuzaim, Abdullah M Alojayri, Fahed A Albednah, Faisal F Alshehri, Mohannad S Alomari, Meshal A Alyousef and Nahaa E Alsubaie,' Impact of Work Hours on the Quality of Life of Adult Employees With Irritable Bowel Syndrome in Saudi Arabia', 28 November 2022, https://www.ncbi.nlm.nih.gov/pmc/articles/PMC9797153/

page 103. 'Moreover, individuals with IBS who experience high levels of anxiety and depression may have suicidal thoughts due to their symptoms, highlighting the severity of the condition...', Mihaela Fadgyas-Stanculete, Ana-Maria Buga, Aurel Popa-Wagner and Dan L Dumitrascu, 'The relationship between irritable bowel syndrome and psychiatric disorders: from molecular changes to clinical manifestations', 27 June 2014, https://www.ncbi.nlm.nih.gov/pmc/articles/PMC4223878/

Chapter 25

page 106. Charles Dickens. "A very little key will open a very heavy door." TheGoldenQuotes.net, https://www.thegoldenquotes.net/best-100-public-domain-quotes-of-all-time-collection-01

page 107. 'Adjusting your diet, taking lactase supplements, which are digestive enzymes, and reducing swallowed air are common methods to reduce gas discomfort...' National Institute of Diabetes and Digestive and Kidney Disease, 'Treatment for Gas in the Digestive Tract', June 2021, https://www.niddk.nih.gov/health-information/digestive-diseases/gas-digestive-tract/treatment

page 108. 'Limit flaxseed powder intake to 2 tablespoons per day accompanied by 150ml of fluid with each tablespoon, and avoid wheat bran...', Wioletta Nowak and Małgorzata Jeziorek, 'The Role of Flaxseed in Improving Human Health', 30 January 2023, https://www.ncbi.nlm.nih.gov/pmc/articles/PMC9914786/

page 108. 'As discussed in the chapter 'Potential Impact of Body Types on IBS', Triphala might help…', Christine Tara Peterson, Kate Denniston and Deepak Chopra, 'Therapeutic Uses of Triphala in Ayurvedic Medicine', 1 August 2017, https://www.ncbi.nlm.nih.gov/pmc/articles/PMC5567597/

page 108. 'Kiwifruit contains 2-3% dietary fibre and is thought to have laxative effects…', Giuseppe Chiarioni, Stefan Lucian Popa, Abdulrahman Ismaiel, Cristina Pop, Dinu Iuliu Dumitrascu, Vlad Dumitru Brata, Traian Adrian Duse, Victor Incze and Teodora Surdea-Blaga, 'Herbal Remedies for Constipation-Predominant Irritable Bowel Syndrome: A Systematic Review of Randomized Controlled Trials', 29 September 2023, https://www.ncbi.nlm.nih.gov/pmc/articles/PMC10574070/

page 110. 'papaya fruit contains papain, an enzyme that supports protein digestion, potentially reducing acid reflux and heartburn…', Yun-Mi Kang, Hyun-Ae Kang, Divina C Cominguez, Su-Hyun Kim and Hyo-Jin An, 'Papain Ameliorates Lipid Accumulation and Inflammation in High-Fat Diet-Induced Obesity Mice and 3T3-L1 Adipocytes via AMPK Activation', 14 September 2021, https://www.ncbi.nlm.nih.gov/pmc/articles/PMC8468764/

page 110. 'According to research published in PubMed Central, fatigue commonly accompanies IBS. IBS involves a breakdown in communication between the gut and the brain, with the Vagus nerve…', Mónica Gros, Belén Gros, José Emilio Mesonero, and Eva Latorre, 'Neurotransmitter Dysfunction in Irritable Bowel Syndrome: Emerging Approaches for Management', 31 July 2021, https://www.ncbi.nlm.nih.gov/pmc/articles/PMC8347293/

page 110. 'For the Vagus nerve to function optimally, your body must be relaxed (parasympathetic)…', Sigrid Breit, Aleksandra Kupferberg, Gerhard Rogler and Gregor Hasler, 'Vagus Nerve as Modulator of the Brain–Gut Axis in Psychiatric and Inflammatory Disorders', 13 March 2018, https://www.ncbi.nlm.nih.gov/pmc/articles/PMC5859128/

page 111. 'Healthy fats, particularly Omega-3s, are essential for brain function, hormonal balance, and managing fatigue…', James J DiNicolantonio and James H O'Keefe, 'The Importance of Marine Omega-3s for Brain Development and the Prevention and Treatment of Behavior, Mood, and Other Brain Disorders', 4 August 2020, https://www.ncbi.nlm.nih.gov/pmc/articles/PMC7468918/

page 111. 'briefly dip your hands in a bowl of ice water for 2 minutes. This can help reduce fatigue in IBS by stimulating…', Dr David Geier, 'Cold exposure: Hands in an ice bucket', 19 July 2019, see https://www.youtube.com/watch?app=desktop&v=Dp5Sp6JJzPM

Chapter 26

page 113. John Barrymore. "Happiness often sneaks in through a door you didn't know you left open." TheGoldenQuotes.net, https://www.thegoldenquotes.net/best-100-public-domain-quotes-of-all-time-collection-01/best-100-public-domain-quotes-of-all-time-collection-03

page 113. Alexandre Dumas. "For all evils there are two remedies - time and silence." TheGoldenQuotes.net, https://www.thegoldenquotes.net/best-100-public-domain-quotes-of-all-time-collection-01/best-100-public-domain-quotes-of-all-time-collection-02

page 113. 'The diverse community of microorganisms that live in the human gut has a wide range of metabolic abilities that complement the functions of enzymes in the liver…', Ian Rowland, Glenn Gibson, Almut Heinken, Karen Scott, Jonathan Swann, Ines Thiele and Kieran Tuohy, 'Gut microbiota functions: metabolism of nutrients and other food components', 9 April 2017, https://www.ncbi.nlm.nih.gov/pmc/articles/PMC5847071/

page 113. 'Researchers are particularly interested in identifying specific microorganisms involved in various metabolic processes, including breaking down dietary carbohydrates into short-chain fatty acids and gases, processing proteins, metabolising plant…', Ian Rowland, Glenn Gibson, Almut Heinken, Karen

References

Scott, Jonathan Swann, Ines Thiele, and Kieran Tuohy, 'Gut microbiota functions: metabolism of nutrients and other food components', 9 April 2017, https://www.ncbi.nlm.nih.gov/pmc/articles/PMC5847071/

page 113. 'IBS is associated with an increase in certain bacteria like Firmicutes, including Ruminococcus, Clostridium, and Dorea, and a decrease in beneficial...', and 'Recent research suggests that microbiome activity and composition differences may influence individual responses to the low FODMAP diet, highlighting the potential for personalised approaches...', Sofia D Shaikh, Natalie Sun, Andrew Canakis, William Y Park and Horst Christian Weber, 'Irritable Bowel Syndrome and the Gut Microbiome: A Comprehensive Review', 28 March 2023, https://www.ncbi.nlm.nih.gov/pmc/articles/PMC10095554/

page 114. 'The polyphenolic profile of cocoa can vary based on the type of cocoa, where it is grown, and how it is processed. The health effects and availability of cocoa polyphenols...', Vincenzo Sorrenti, Sawan Ali, Laura Mancin, Sergio Davinelli, Antonio Paoli, and Giovanni Scapagnini, 'Cocoa Polyphenols and Gut Microbiota Interplay: Bioavailability, Prebiotic Effect, and Impact on Human Health', 27 June 2020, https://www.ncbi.nlm.nih.gov/pmc/articles/PMC7400387/

page 114. 'Urbanisation and soil degradation likely impact the composition of gut microbes, potentially increasing bacteria associated with dysbiosis, such as Proteobacteria...', Nishat Tasnim, Nijiati Abulizi, Jason Pither, Miranda M Hart, and Deanna L. Gibson, 'Linking the Gut Microbial Ecosystem with the Environment: Does Gut Health Depend on Where We Live?', 6 October 2017, https://www.ncbi.nlm.nih.gov/pmc/articles/PMC5635058/

page 114. 'A study across 1,044 participants revealed that regular exercise leads to a notable increase...', Leizi Min, Alimjan Ablitip, Rui Wang, Torquati Luciana, Mengxian Wei, and Xindong Ma, 'Effects of Exercise on Gut Microbiota of Adults: A Systematic Review and Meta-Analysis', 5 April 2024, https://www.ncbi.nlm.nih.gov/pmc/articles/PMC11013040/

page 115. 'Research suggests a U-shaped relationship where 7 hours of sleep per night is optimal. Sleeping less or more than 7 hours increases the risk of metabolic syndrome, including obesity...', Jingyi Sun, Dan Fang, Zhiqiang Wang, and Yuan Liu, 'Sleep Deprivation and Gut Microbiota Dysbiosis: Current Understandings and Implications', 31 May 2023, https://www.ncbi.nlm.nih.gov/pmc/articles/PMC10253795/

page 115. 'Research shows that chronic stress alters the composition of gut microbes, reducing beneficial bacteria and increasing harmful ones...', Alison Warren, Yvonne Nyavor, Aaron Beguelin and Leigh A Frame, 'Dangers of the chronic stress response in the context of the microbiota-gut-immune-brain axis and mental health: a narrative review', 2 May 2024, https://www.ncbi.nlm.nih.gov/pmc/articles/PMC11096445/

page 115. 'The relationship between gut microbiota (GM), ageing, and longevity has become increasingly clear in recent years, highlighting its significant impact on how we age. Various factors affect...', Juan Salazar, Pablo Durán, María P Díaz, Maricarmen Chacín, Raquel Santeliz, Edgardo Mengual, Emma Gutiérrez, Xavier León, Andrea Díaz, Marycarlota Bernal, Daniel Escalona, Luis Alberto Parra Hernández, and Valmore Bermúdez, 'Exploring the Relationship between the Gut Microbiota and Ageing: A Possible Age Modulato', 17 May 2023, https://www.ncbi.nlm.nih.gov/pmc/articles/PMC10218639/

page 115. 'Saliva samples were collected from 846 women and 368 men aged 35–69 years participating in the Atlantic Partnership for Tomorrow's Health (PATH), a Canadian population...', Vanessa DeClercq, Jacob T Nearing and Morgan G I Langille, 'Investigation of the impact of commonly used medications on the oral microbiome of individuals living without major chronic conditions', 9 December 2021, https://www.ncbi.nlm.nih.gov/pmc/articles/PMC8659300/

Chapter 27

page 118. Blaise Pascal. "Don't try to add more years to your life. Better add more life to your years." TheGoldenQuotes.net, https://www.thegoldenquotes.net/best-100-public-domain-quotes-of-all-time-collection-01/best-100-public-domain-quotes-of-all-time-collection-02

page 118. 'There is growing interest in altering the microbiome to prevent or treat illnesses, leading to the development of various strategies. However, progress is slowed by uncertainties about the precise…', Eamonn M M Quigley and Prianka Gajula, 'Recent advances in modulating the microbiome', 27 January 2020, https://www.ncbi.nlm.nih.gov/pmc/articles/PMC6993818/

page 118. 'During the 2010s, interest in the gut microbiome surged in life sciences research and industry, leading Forbes to name it "The Decade of the Microbiome." This rise was…', Janet M Sasso, Ramy M Ammar, Rumiana Tenchov, Steven Lemmel, Olaf Kelber, Malte Grieswelle and Qiongqiong Angela Zhou, 'Gut Microbiome–Brain Alliance: A Landscape View into Mental and Gastrointestinal Health and Disorders', 8 May 2023, https://www.ncbi.nlm.nih.gov/pmc/articles/PMC10197139/

page 118. 'FMT involves transferring stool from a healthy donor into the gut…', Dana Al-Ali, Aamena Ahmed, Ameena Shafiq, Clare McVeigh, Ali Chaari, Dalia Zakaria, and Ghizlane Bendriss, 'Fecal microbiota transplants: A review of emerging clinical data on applications, efficacy, and risks (2015–2020)', 22 February 2021, https://www.ncbi.nlm.nih.gov/pmc/articles/PMC8475724/

page 119. 'Metabolomics has identified specific substances, like THDOC in the blood linked to depression, that show significant differences between individuals with…', Lijuan Han, Ling Zhao, Yong Zhou, Chao Yang, Teng Xiong, Lin Lu, Yusheng Deng, Wen Luo, Yang Chen, Qinwei Qiu, Xiaoxiao Shang, Li Huang, Zongchao Mo, Shaogang Huang, Suiping Huang, Zhi Liu, Wei Yang, Lixiang Zhai, Ziwan Ning, Chengyuan Lin, Tao Huang, Chungwah Cheng, Linda L D Zhong, Shuaicheng Li, Zhaoxiang Bian and Xiaodong Fang, 'Altered metabolome and microbiome features provide clues in understanding irritable bowel syndrome and depression comorbidity', 8 November 2021, https://www.ncbi.nlm.nih.gov/pmc/articles/PMC8940891/

page 119. 'The study explored two main themes: critical metabolites linked to IBS and dietary interventions to reduce symptoms and severity of IBS. While clinical studies on reducing…', Shanalee C James, Karl Fraser, Wayne Young, Warren C McNabb and Nicole C, 'Gut Microbial Metabolites and Biochemical Pathways Involved in Irritable Bowel Syndrome: Effects of Diet and Nutrition on the Microbiome', 31 December 2019, https://www.ncbi.nlm.nih.gov/pmc/articles/PMC7198292/

page 119. 'Using advanced technologies like genomics, transcriptomics, and proteomics to tailor treatment plans based on each person's gut microbiome is an exciting medical frontier…', Claudia Manzoni, Demis A Kia, Jana Vandrovcova, John Hardy, Nicholas W Wood, Patrick A Lewis and Raffaele Ferrari, 'Genome, transcriptome and proteome: the rise of omics data and their integration in biomedical sciences', 22 November 2016, https://www.ncbi.nlm.nih.gov/pmc/articles/PMC6018996/

page 120. 'The variety of sequencing and bioinformatics methods available can produce varied results, highlighting the need for a systematic approach…', Jingyue Wu, Stephanie S Singleton, Urnisha Bhuiyan, Lori Krammer and Raja Mazumder, 'ulti-omics approaches to studying gastrointestinal microbiome in the context of precision medicine and machine learning', 19 January 2024, https://www.ncbi.nlm.nih.gov/pmc/articles/PMC10834744/

page 120. ' 'There are concerns about increasing human reliance on machines, potentially reducing our ability to perform tasks independently. However, it is essential to acknowledge that technology enhances efficiency and maintains high standards…', Radu Alexandru Vulpoi, Mihaela Luca, Adrian Ciobanu, Andrei Olteanu, Oana Bărboi, Diana-Elena Iov, Loredana Nichita, Irina Ciortescu, Cristina Cijevschi Prelipcean, Gabriela Ștefănescu, Cătălina Mihai and Vasile Liviu Drug, 'The Potential Use of Artificial Intelligence in Irritable Bowel Syndrome Management', 29 October 2023, https://www.ncbi.nlm.nih.gov/pmc/articles/PMC10648815/

References

page 120. 'Research suggests that postbiotics could offer a new approach to treating IBS by…', Linxi Ma, Huaijun Tu and Tingtao Chen, 'Postbiotics in Human Health: A Narrative Review', 6 January 2023, https://www.ncbi.nlm.nih.gov/pmc/articles/PMC9863882/

page 121. 'The study looked at different types of gastrointestinal (GI) cancers. They found that microbial profiles…', Jihan Wang , Yangyang Wang , Zhenzhen Li, Xiaoguang Gao and Dageng Huang , 'Global Analysis of Microbiota Signatures in Four Major Types of Gastrointestinal Cancer', 5 August 2021, https://www.ncbi.nlm.nih.gov/pmc/articles/PMC8375155/

page 121. 'A study pointed out significant variations in metabolites among individuals with IBS. Metabolites are small molecules that play critical roles in various biological processes within the body, making…', Lin Xiao, Qin Liu, Mei Luo and Lishou Xiong, 'Gut Microbiota-Derived Metabolites in Irritable Bowel Syndrome', 23 September 2021, https://www.ncbi.nlm.nih.gov/pmc/articles/PMC8495119/

page 122. 'Moreover, the study revealed that combining medications with antipsychotic medications may promote the growth of beneficial bacteria like Akkermansia muciniphila, positively affecting metabolism and insulin sensitivity (Depommier et al., 2019)…', Agata Misera, Igor Łoniewski, Joanna Palma, Monika Kulaszyńska, Wiktoria Czarnecka, Mariusz Kaczmarczyk, Paweł Liśkiewicz, Jerzy Samochowiec and Karolina Skonieczna-Żydecka, 'Clinical significance of microbiota changes under the influence of psychotropic drugs. An updated narrative review', 1 March 2023, https://www.ncbi.nlm.nih.gov/pmc/articles/PMC10014913/

page 122. 'The research indicates that while SSRIs and therapies aimed at improving bowel movements benefit specific individuals, they advocate for a comprehensive…', Emeran A Mayer, Hyo Jin Ryu and Ravi R. Bhatt, 'The neurobiology of irritable bowel syndrome', 2 February 2023, https://www.ncbi.nlm.nih.gov/pmc/articles/PMC10208985/

page 122. 'Many individuals with IBS have imbalances in their gut bacteria, which are closely linked to when their symptoms start and how severe they are. While probiotics have shown some promise in treating IBS, researchers…', Minjia Chen, Guangcong Ruan, Lu Chen, Senhong Ying, Guanhu Li, Fenghua Xu, Zhifeng Xiao, Yuting Tian, Linling Lv, Yi Ping, Yi Cheng and Yanling Wei, 'Neurotransmitter and Intestinal Interactions: Focus on the Microbiota-Gut-Brain Axis in Irritable Bowel Syndrome',16 February 2022, https://www.ncbi.nlm.nih.gov/pmc/articles/PMC8888441/

page 123. 'By closely examining how stress, genetics, epigenetics, and gut bacteria affect IBS, researchers aim to better understand its causes. This could lead to new tests…', Swapna Mahurkar-Joshi and Lin Chang, 'Epigenetic Mechanisms in Irritable Bowel Syndrome', 14 August 2020, https://www.ncbi.nlm.nih.gov/pmc/articles/PMC7456856/

page 124. 'Researchers understanding of gut bacteria has improved, and the findings suggested they also need to study other microbes like viruses and eukaryotes. For instance…', Ronald D Hills Jr., Benjamin A Pontefract, Hillary R Mishcon, Cody A Black, Steven C Sutton and Cory R Theberge, 'Gut Microbiome: Profound Implications for Diet and Disease', 16 July 2019, https://www.ncbi.nlm.nih.gov/pmc/articles/PMC6682904/

page 124. 'The research says using specially engineered bacteria is one advanced way to improve microbiome health. Unlike regular probiotics, these bacteria are designed to…', Nikhil Aggarwal, Shohei Kitano, Ginette Ru Ying Puah, Sandra Kittelmann, In Young Hwang and Matthew Wook Chang, 'Microbiome and Human Health: Current Understanding, Engineering, and Enabling Technologies', 1 November 2022, https://www.ncbi.nlm.nih.gov/pmc/articles/PMC9837825/

page 124. 'The research approach involved using the Blueprint persona method with a focus group of experts from various fields to identify the need for a mobile health (mHealth) intervention…', Maurizio Gentile, Vincenzo De Luca, Roberta Patalano, Daniela Laudisio, Giovanni Tramontano, Sonja Lindner-Rabl, Lorenzo Mercurio, Elena Salvatore, John Farrell, Regina Roller-Wirnsberger, Lutz Kubitschke,

Maria Triassi, Annamaria Colao, Maddalena Illario and Vigour Consortium, 'Innovative approaches to service integration addressing the unmet needs of irritable bowel syndrome patients and new approaches for the needs of IBS patients', 16 November 2022, https://www.ncbi.nlm.nih.gov/pmc/articles/PMC9709639/

page 125. 'Studies suggest there might be a link between gut bacteria and autoimmune conditions such as Rheumatoid arthritis, multiple sclerosis...', Yu Zhang, Jiazhi Liao and Wenjuan Fan, 'Role of autoantibodies in the pathophysiology of irritable bowel syndrome: a review', 5 March 2024, https://www.ncbi.nlm.nih.gov/pmc/articles/PMC10948515/

Final Thoughts

page 129. Oscar Wilde. "The well bred contradict other people. The wise contradict themselves." TheGoldenQuotes.net, https://www.thegoldenquotes.net/best-100-public-domain-quotes-of-all-time-collection-01/best-100-public-domain-quotes-of-all-time-collection-04

page 129. Original image by Ninikvaratskhelia. Edited by Jan Nallathamby. "John Lennon once shared a piece of wisdom from his grandmother: "Never say you are sick. Even if you are sick. Say you are healing. Words do manifest." https://pixabay.com/illustrations/grandmother-love-girl-happy-7427525/

Disclaimer: the organisations cited in the academic research articles above are not affiliated with this book.

Index

A